# DBT Mastery for Alcohol Recovery

Navigating Triggers and Emotional
Regulation for Sustained Sobriety

Billy Wilsfriend

# Contents

# Preface

The sun had barely risen, casting a soft orange hue over the city. In a small apartment on the 15th floor, Mark sat on his balcony, a cup of coffee in hand. But instead of savoring the morning calm, his mind was racing, trapped in a relentless cycle of regret and what-ifs. Just the night before, he had promised himself, "Tonight's the last time." Yet, here he was, nursing a hangover, the empty bottles from the previous night serving as a stark reminder of his broken promise.

It's said that the definition of insanity is doing the same thing over and over again and expecting different results. If that's true, then many of us are caught in our own loops of madness, repeating patterns we despise, yet feeling powerless to change. It's like being stuck in a maze, knowing there's an exit, but every turn seems to lead to another dead end.

Have you ever felt trapped in your own life? As if you're watching a movie where the protagonist keeps making the same mistakes, and you're shouting at the screen, hoping they'd choose differently, only to realize that the protagonist is you? The weight of such realization can be crushing. It's the weight of missed opportunities, of relationships strained, of potential unfulfilled. It's the silent scream in the middle of the night, the tear that slips when no one's watching, the heavy sigh that says, "I wish things were different."

But what if they could be? Imagine a life where the chains that once held you back are broken. A life where you wake up with a sense of purpose, where your past doesn't dictate your future, and where every new day is a blank canvas, waiting for you to paint your masterpiece. Can you feel the exhilaration of freedom, the joy of rediscovery, the warmth of genuine connections?

This isn't just a flight of fancy. It's a glimpse into a reality that's within your grasp. A reality where you're not just surviving, but thriving. Where every challenge is an opportunity, every setback a lesson, and every success a stepping stone to even greater heights.

Hold onto that vision. Let it be the beacon that guides you through the storm, the anchor that grounds you, and the wind that propels you forward. Because no matter how dark the night, dawn always follows. And with it comes the promise of a new beginning.

In the vast sea of literature, there are countless books that promise solutions, change, and transformation. But what sets this journey apart? Why is this narrative any different? The answer is simple: this isn't just a book; it's a compass, a guide, a mentor, and a friend. It's a beacon in the darkest nights and a map for the most treacherous terrains.

You're about to delve into a world that marries time-tested wisdom with groundbreaking insights. A world where every page is a step closer to the life you've always envisioned. Here, you'll uncover:

- Strategies that aren't mere theories but are born from real-life experiences and challenges.

- Techniques that have been refined over time, ensuring they're not just effective but also adaptable to your unique journey.

- Stories that aren't just tales but mirrors reflecting shared human experiences, struggles, and triumphs.

While many books offer a one-size-fits-all approach, this narrative recognizes and celebrates your individuality. It doesn't just offer solutions; it empowers you to create your own. It's not about following a script; it's about writing your own story.

You might wonder, "Who is behind these words? Why should I trust this voice?" Let me share a bit of my journey with you.

Years ago, I stood at a crossroads, much like Mark from our story. The weight of my choices, both good and bad, bore down on me. It was during these trying times that I stumbled upon the principles and techniques you'll find in these pages. They weren't just theories in textbooks; they were lifelines that pulled me from the depths of despair.

My passion for this subject isn't academic; it's deeply personal. Every word penned here is a piece of my heart, a fragment of my soul. I've walked the path, faced the storms, and basked in the sunshine that follows. And now, I'm here to walk beside you, ensuring you never feel alone in your journey.

My commitment isn't just to share knowledge but to be a testament to its power. To show that if someone like me, with all my flaws and failures, can find a way, so can you.

As we transition from this introduction to the heart of our narrative, remember this: every chapter, every page, every word is a step. Some steps might be challenging, others enlightening, but each one is essential. This isn't a sprint; it's a marathon. And like any marathon, it's not just about the destination but the journey itself.

Expect moments of introspection, bursts of revelation, and periods of contemplation. There will be times when you'll want to pause, reflect, and maybe even reread. That's okay. This journey is yours, and you set the pace.

So, as you turn the page, know that you're not just reading a book. You're embarking on a transformative journey, one that promises not just change but evolution. A journey where every challenge faced is a lesson learned, every setback an opportunity for growth, and every success a testament to your resilience.

Hold tight to the vision we painted earlier. Let it guide you, inspire you, and remind you of the potential that lies within. Because this journey, your journey, is just beginning.

# Introduction

Imagine standing at the edge of a vast ocean, the waves crashing against the shore, representing the tumultuous emotions and challenges of alcoholism. You want to cross it, to reach the serene island of recovery on the other side. But how? This chapter is your boat, designed to navigate the turbulent waters of alcoholism using the principles of DBT.

In this chapter, we'll embark on a journey to understand the profound impact of DBT in the realm of alcohol recovery. We'll delve deep into the comprehensive knowledge of DBT, explore practical tools and techniques tailored for alcoholism, and discover pathways to personal growth and mending relationships.

The story of DBT and alcoholism is akin to a master locksmith crafting the perfect key for a particularly tricky lock. Alcoholism, with its intricate challenges and deeply rooted issues, is that lock. And DBT? It's the meticulously crafted key.

Imagine for a moment a library. This isn't any ordinary library, but one that holds the secrets of the human mind. In one of its quiet corners, there's a book titled "DBT: The Master Key." As you open it, the first chapter reads, "Comprehensive Knowledge."

DBT, or Dialectical Behavior Therapy, wasn't initially designed for alcoholism. Its roots trace back to treating borderline personality disorder. But like any great story, there was an unexpected twist. Clinicians began to notice its potential for treating a range of other issues, including alcoholism. It's like discovering that a melody crafted for a violin sounds even more enchanting on a piano.

As you turn the pages of this metaphorical book, you come across tales of individuals, much like Mark from our earlier narrative, who found solace in the principles of DBT. Their stories aren't just about abstaining from alcohol but about rediscovering themselves, mending broken relationships, and charting a course to a brighter future.

But how does DBT achieve this? Imagine a toolkit. Not the kind filled with hammers and nails, but one brimming with strategies, exercises, and techniques. This is the "Practical Tools and Techniques" section of our DBT book.

One of the most powerful tools in this kit is mindfulness. Picture yourself in a bustling market, surrounded by the cacophony of vendors, shoppers, and the general hustle and bustle. Amidst this chaos, you're trying to listen to a soft tune playing somewhere in the distance. Mindfulness is the act of tuning out the noise and focusing solely on that melody. In the context of alcoholism, it's about recognizing triggers, understanding emotions, and making conscious choices.

Another chapter in this section might be titled "Emotional Regulation." Think of it as learning to dance in the rain instead of waiting for the storm to pass. It's about embracing emotions, understanding them, and channeling them in a positive direction.

As we delve deeper, we encounter the chapter on "Personal Growth and Relationship Repair." Alcoholism doesn't just affect the individual; it sends ripples through their entire circle, straining relationships and trust.

Imagine a tapestry, once vibrant and intact, now torn and frayed due to the wear and tear of time and neglect. DBT acts as the skilled craftsman, meticulously mending each tear, restoring the tapestry to its former glory. It offers strategies to rebuild trust, foster open communication, and heal wounds, both old and new.

But it's not just about mending what's broken. It's about adding new threads, weaving new stories, and creating a tapestry that's even more beautiful than before.

The journey through the world of DBT and alcoholism is profound and transformative. It offers a beacon of hope to those lost in the stormy seas of addiction. Some of the most pivotal revelations from this chapter include:

- DBT's Versatility: Originally designed for a different purpose, DBT has shown remarkable efficacy in treating alcoholism, proving that solutions can often come from the most unexpected places.

- Mindfulness as a Superpower: In a world filled with distractions, the ability to focus, to truly be present, is invaluable. Mindfulness isn't just a tool; it's a way of life.

- Embracing Emotions: Instead of shunning or fearing emotions, DBT teaches us to embrace them. It's about understanding that emotions aren't the enemy; it's our reaction to them that determines the outcome.

- The Ripple Effect: Alcoholism doesn't exist in isolation. It affects every facet of an individual's life. But with the right tools and strategies, it's possible to mend broken relationships and chart a course to personal growth.

Imagine standing at the threshold of a grand mansion, having only explored its majestic entrance. The rooms beyond beckon with promises of untold stories, hidden treasures, and profound wisdom. This chapter was that entrance, a mere glimpse into the vast expanse of knowledge and insights that DBT offers. As we stand at this juncture, let's take a moment to reflect and prepare for the deeper exploration that lies ahead.

Think of DBT as a symphony, a harmonious blend of various instruments, each playing its unique role. We've just listened to the opening notes, resonating with promise and hope. But a symphony isn't just about its beginning; it's the crescendos, the quiet moments, the transitions, and the finale that make it complete.

In the upcoming sections, we'll delve into each 'instrument' of DBT. We'll understand how they come together to create a melody that has the power to heal, transform, and inspire.

One of the core principles of DBT is the concept of dialectics. It's the art of balancing opposites, of finding harmony amidst contradictions. Imagine a tightrope walker, gracefully balancing on a thin wire, with vast chasms on either side. On one side is acceptance, and on the other, change. The tightrope walker's skill lies in navigating this delicate balance, ensuring neither side outweighs the other. In our journey through DBT, we'll learn how to be that tightrope walker, mastering the dance of dialectics.

Another cornerstone of DBT is the emphasis on being present. In today's fast-paced world, our minds are often scattered, juggling past regrets and future anxieties. But true healing, true transformation, lies in the power of now. Picture a serene lake, its waters still, reflecting the world around it with crystal clarity. When we learn to be present, our minds become like that lake, calm, clear, and reflective. We'll delve deeper into techniques and exercises that help us harness this power, enabling us to live each moment to its fullest.

At its core, DBT is not just about recovery from alcoholism; it's a journey of self-discovery. It's about understanding oneself, recognizing patterns, and reshaping narratives. Imagine standing in front of a mirror, but instead of reflecting your physical self, it reveals your thoughts, emotions, and innermost desires. Through DBT, we'll learn to look into this mirror, to confront our reflections, and to embark on a transformative journey of self-awareness and growth.

As we prepare to delve deeper into this world of DBT, remember that this is a journey, not a destination. It's about the insights gained, the challenges overcome, and the transformations experienced along the way. So, with an open heart and a curious mind, let's continue our exploration, hand in hand, step by step, into the heart of DBT and its profound impact on alcohol recovery. The next chapter awaits, filled with more stories, strategies, and revelations, all designed to guide, inspire, and empower.

# Chapter One

---

# The Essence of DBT: Foundations and Principles

"In this world of black and white, it's our ability to weave through the grays that counts. And that's the essence of DBT." - Marsha Linehan, the founder of DBT.

In this chapter, we embark on a journey through the intricate tapestry of Dialectical Behavior Therapy (DBT). From its historical roots to its core principles, and its profound significance in alcohol recovery, we'll delve deep, unraveling the transformative power of DBT.

The late 20th century was a time of rapid evolution in the realm of psychotherapy. Amidst this evolution, DBT emerged as a beacon of hope for those grappling with intense emotional pain, particularly individuals with borderline personality disorder. The therapy, while rooted in cognitive behavioral therapy, introduced a fresh perspective, emphasizing the balance between acceptance and change.

Marsha Linehan wasn't just the founder of DBT; she was its heart and soul. Her personal struggles with mental health provided her with insights that went beyond textbooks. She envisioned a therapy that was compassionate, holistic, and deeply transformative. DBT was her brainchild, a therapy that seamlessly blended cognitive-behavioral techniques with the age-old wisdom of mindfulness.

DBT's principles, while universal, found a unique application in the realm of alcohol recovery. The therapy's emphasis on emotional regulation, distress tolerance, and interpersonal effectiveness provided individuals battling alcoholism with tools that were both practical and profound.

Consider the story of Alex, a 35-year-old battling the demons of alcoholism. Traditional therapies provided temporary relief but didn't address the core issues. Enter DBT, and the transformation was palpable. Through DBT, Alex learned to navigate emotional upheavals, build meaningful relationships, and most importantly, believe in the possibility of a life free from the shackles of alcohol.

At the heart of DBT lies the principle of mindfulness. It's not just a technique; it's a way of life. Mindfulness is about being present, fully and completely. For someone battling alcoholism, this presence becomes their anchor, allowing them to navigate the tumultuous seas of cravings and relapses with clarity and conviction.

Emotions, in their raw intensity, can often become overwhelming. DBT, through its emphasis on emotional regulation, provides individuals with tools to understand, express, and manage their emotions. It's not about suppression; it's about expression, in ways that are healthy and healing.

Life is unpredictable, filled with highs and lows. Distress tolerance is about navigating these lows with resilience. It's about facing challenges head-on, without resorting to unhealthy coping mechanisms like alcohol.

Relationships play a pivotal role in our lives. DBT, through its focus on interpersonal effectiveness, empowers individuals to build and nurture relationships that are meaningful and fulfilling. It's about communication, boundaries, and mutual respect.

In the vast landscape of therapies for alcohol recovery, DBT stands out, not just in its approach but in its results. While most therapies focus on the past, DBT emphasizes the present, equipping individuals with tools to navigate their current challenges.

DBT isn't just a therapeutic approach; it's a science-backed intervention. Research has consistently highlighted the efficacy of DBT in addressing the multifaceted challenges of addiction. The therapy, with its emphasis on mindfulness, emotional regulation, and interpersonal effectiveness, addresses the root causes of addiction, facilitating deep and lasting transformation.

Every individual's journey with alcoholism is unique. DBT recognizes this uniqueness and tailors its interventions accordingly. Through personalized strategies and interventions, DBT ensures that the therapy aligns with the individual's challenges, aspirations, and recovery goals.

The term 'dialectical' might sound complex, but its essence is simple: it's about balance. At its core, DBT emphasizes the reconciliation of opposites, the harmonizing of acceptance and change. This balance is crucial, especially for those battling alcoholism. On one hand, there's the need to accept one's current state, the reality of addiction. On the other, there's the burning desire for change, for a life free from the chains of alcohol. DBT beautifully bridges these seemingly opposing forces, creating a path of holistic healing.

Imagine being on a boat, with turbulent waves on one side and calm waters on the other. The turbulent waves represent the chaos of addiction, the emotional upheavals, the broken promises. The calm waters symbolize hope, the possibility of a life of sobriety and serenity. DBT is like the skilled sailor who knows when to let the boat ride the waves and when to steer it towards calmer waters. It's this dance between acceptance and change that makes DBT so transformative.

Validation is a cornerstone of DBT. It's about acknowledging one's feelings, experiences, and challenges without judgment. For someone battling alcoholism, this validation can be profoundly healing. It's a balm for the soul, a gentle reminder that one's feelings are valid, that the pain is real, but so is the possibility of healing. Through validation, DBT creates a therapeutic environment where individuals feel seen, heard, and understood.

DBT isn't a one-size-fits-all approach. It's structured, yet flexible, tailored to the unique needs of the individual. Typically, DBT involves individual therapy sessions, where deep-seated issues are addressed, and group sessions, where skills are learned and practiced. These sessions are like the two wings of a bird, each crucial for the therapeutic journey.

DBT is as much about insight as it is about action. The therapy emphasizes skills training, equipping individuals with practical tools to navigate the challenges of life. These skills are broadly categorized into

four modules: Mindfulness, Emotional Regulation, Distress Tolerance, and Interpersonal Effectiveness. Each module is a treasure trove
of strategies, exercises, and interventions, designed to empower individuals to live a life of balance, purpose, and joy.

In DBT, the therapist isn't just a passive listener; they're an active
participant in the therapeutic journey. They're the guide, the mentor,
the anchor. They challenge, support, validate, and inspire. Their role
is multifaceted, ranging from teaching skills and providing feedback to
creating a safe space where individuals can explore their vulnerabilities
and strengths.

DBT isn't confined to the four walls of the therapy room. Its principles
are universal, applicable to the myriad challenges of daily life. Whether
it's navigating a difficult conversation, dealing with a setback, or simply being present in the moment, DBT offers insights and tools that
are both practical and profound.

Recovery isn't a destination; it's a journey, a lifelong journey. And
DBT is a constant companion on this journey. The skills learned in
DBT aren't just for the challenging times; they're for life. They're the
compass that guides, the anchor that grounds, and the wings that
empower individuals to soar to new heights.

Mindfulness, at its core, is about being present. It's about fully immersing oneself in the current moment, free from the shackles of the
past and the anxieties of the future. In the context of DBT, mindfulness is more than just a meditative practice; it's a way of life. It's
the foundation upon which all other skills are built, the bedrock of
self-awareness and self-regulation.

Imagine standing at the edge of a serene lake, the water's surface perfectly still, reflecting the azure sky above. Now, imagine throwing a stone into the lake. The ripples spread outwards, disturbing the tranquility of the water. Our minds are much like that lake. Thoughts, emotions, and external stimuli constantly create ripples, disturbing our inner peace. Mindfulness is the act of observing these ripples without judgment, of being a silent witness to the ebb and flow of our inner world. It's about returning to the breath, the anchor that grounds us in the present moment.

While the practice of mindfulness often conjures images of serene meditation sessions, in DBT, it's as much about action as it is about stillness. It's about being mindful in everyday activities, whether it's savoring a meal, listening to a loved one, or simply taking a walk. It's about fully engaging with life, moment by moment, with a sense of curiosity and wonder.

Our emotions are like a vast landscape, with towering mountains, deep valleys, serene meadows, and turbulent storms. They add color, depth, and richness to our lives. However, for someone grappling with alcoholism, this landscape can often feel overwhelming, un-predictable, and treacherous. DBT offers the tools and strategies to navigate this landscape with skill, grace, and resilience.

Emotions, in their essence, are neutral. They are neither good nor bad; they simply are. They play a dual role in our lives: they inform and they motivate. They inform us about our inner world, our needs, desires, and boundaries. They motivate us to take action, to move towards pleasure and away from pain. However, when not regulated, emotions can become tyrants, dictating our actions and leading us astray.

Emotional regulation is both an art and a science. It's an art because it requires creativity, intuition, and finesse. It's a science because it's rooted in evidence-based strategies and techniques. In DBT, emotional regulation isn't about suppressing or denying emotions; it's about understanding, accepting, and modulating them. It's about creating a harmonious symphony from the cacophony of our feelings.

Life, with all its beauty and wonder, is also fraught with challenges, setbacks, and distress. For someone on the path of recovery, these distressing moments can be triggers, leading them back into the abyss of addiction. Distress tolerance in DBT is about building resilience, about facing the storms of life with courage, strength, and equanimity.

There's a profound difference between resignation and acceptance. Resignation is passive; it's about giving up. Acceptance, on the other hand, is active; it's about facing reality with an open heart and an open mind. In DBT, acceptance is a powerful tool, a beacon of hope in the darkest of times. It's about acknowledging the pain, the challenge, the distress, without being overwhelmed by it.

Distress tolerance in DBT is not just about acceptance; it's also about action. It's about building a toolkit of strategies, techniques, and interventions to navigate distressing situations. Whether it's deep breathing, grounding exercises, or cognitive reframing, each tool is designed to empower the individual, to give them a sense of agency and control in the face of distress.

As we delve deeper into the intricacies of DBT, let's remember that this journey is not just about acquiring skills; it's about transformation. It's about metamorphosis, about emerging from the cocoon of addiction as a vibrant butterfly, ready to soar to new heights. The path ahead is filled with insights, revelations, and profound transformations. So, let's embark on this journey with an open heart, an open mind, and a spirit of discovery.

### *Mental Notes to Take Into Following Chapters:*

The world of Dialectical Behavior Therapy (DBT) is vast, intricate, and profoundly transformative. As we journeyed through the chapter, we unearthed the foundational pillars of DBT and its profound implications for alcohol recovery. Let's revisit the essence of what we've learned.

The Legacy of Marsha Linehan:

DBT isn't just a therapeutic approach; it's a legacy, a testament to the pioneering work of Marsha Linehan. Her personal and professional journey has illuminated the path for countless individuals, offering hope, healing, and transformation.

DBT's Historical Tapestry:

The history of DBT is a tapestry woven with threads of innovation, adaptation, and evolution. From its origins as a therapy for borderline personality disorder to its adaptation for alcohol recovery, DBT has proven its versatility and efficacy time and again.

The Four Pillars of DBT:

DBT stands tall on four pillars: Mindfulness, Emotional Regulation, Distress Tolerance, and Interpersonal Effectiveness. Each pillar is a beacon of hope, offering tools, strategies, and insights for holistic healing.

- Mindfulness: The art of being present, of fully immersing oneself in the here and now. It's the anchor that grounds us, the compass that guides us, and the sanctuary that offers solace.

- Emotional Regulation: Our emotions are the colors of our inner world. DBT teaches us to paint with these colors, to create a masterpiece of harmony, balance, and resonance.

- Distress Tolerance: Life's storms are inevitable. DBT equips us with the tools to face these storms with resilience, courage, and equanimity.

- Interpersonal Effectiveness: Relationships are the tapestry of our lives. DBT offers the threads to weave this tapestry with love, understanding, and connection.

DBT and Alcohol Recovery:

DBT isn't just another therapy; it's a revolution in the realm of alcohol recovery. It offers a nuanced, holistic, and evidence-based approach, addressing not just the symptoms but the root causes of addiction. By tailoring its strategies and interventions to the unique challenges of alcoholism, DBT offers a beacon of hope to those trapped in the abyss of addiction.

The Transformative Power of DBT:

Transformation is the essence of DBT. It's about metamorphosis, about emerging from the cocoon of pain, suffering, and addiction as a vibrant butterfly, ready to soar to new heights. It's about rediscovering oneself, reclaiming one's power, and rewriting one's story.

The Synergy of DBT's Components:

The beauty of DBT lies not just in its individual components but in their synergy. Each element, from mindfulness to interpersonal effectiveness, doesn't operate in isolation. They intertwine, creating a harmonious dance of healing, growth, and transformation. This synergy amplifies the impact of DBT, making it a holistic and comprehensive approach to healing.

The Science Behind DBT:

DBT isn't just a collection of philosophical insights or therapeutic interventions. It's grounded in rigorous scientific research. Studies have consistently shown the efficacy of DBT in treating a range of disorders, including alcoholism. This scientific foundation lends credibility to DBT, assuring those on the path of recovery that they're in safe, evidence-based hands.

DBT's Unique Approach to Alcohol Recovery:

While there are myriad therapies and interventions for alcohol recovery, DBT stands out with its unique approach. It doesn't just address the act of drinking. It delves deeper, addressing the emotional, psychological, and interpersonal triggers that often lead to relapse. By equipping individuals with tools to manage these triggers, DBT offers a sustainable, long-term approach to recovery.

The Role of Case Studies in DBT:

Throughout our exploration, we encountered various case studies, real-life stories of individuals who've transformed their lives with DBT. These aren't just stories; they're testimonies, powerful reminders of the transformative potential of DBT. They inspire hope, offering tangible proof that change is possible, no matter how deep the abyss of addiction.

DBT's Broader Implications:

While our focus has been on alcohol recovery, it's essential to recognize the broader implications of DBT. Its principles, from mindfulness to emotional regulation, have universal relevance. They offer insights and tools for anyone seeking to lead a more balanced, harmonious, and fulfilling life.

As we stand at this juncture, reflecting on the profound insights and revelations of this chapter, let's take a moment to breathe, to internalize, and to prepare. The path ahead is filled with more discoveries, deeper explorations, and transformative experiences. Our journey with DBT is like a river, flowing seamlessly from one chapter to the next, from one revelation to another. Throughout our exploration, we encountered various case studies, real-life stories of individuals who've transformed their lives with DBT. These aren't just stories; they're testimonies, powerful reminders of the transformative potential of DBT. They inspire hope, offering tangible proof that change is possible, no matter how deep the abyss of addiction. As we prepare to dive into the next chapter, let's carry with us the wisdom, insights, and tools we've gathered, using them as a foundation to build upon, explore, and transform. The adventure continues, and the next chapter promises to be as enlightening and transformative as this one.

# Chapter Two

---

# Recognizing and Navigating Triggers

D id you know that nearly 60% of individuals in recovery from alcohol addiction experience at least one relapse within the first year? This staggering statistic underscores the power and persistence of triggers in the recovery journey.

In this chapter, we'll delve deep into the realm of triggers, understanding their nature, and the pivotal role they play in the recovery process. We'll explore the DBT approach to recognizing and navigating these triggers and the strategies to build resilience against them.

Triggers are akin to silent alarms, often unnoticed but powerful enough to set off a cascade of emotions and reactions. They can be as blatant as a bar's neon sign or as subtle as a particular scent, a song, or even a memory. Let's break down the concept of triggers:

At its core, a trigger is any stimulus that evokes the desire or craving to consume alcohol. It's the whisper in the ear, the nudge towards the bottle. But why are they so crucial? Because understanding triggers is the first step in mastering them. By recognizing what sets off the urge, one can develop strategies to counteract or avoid them.

Triggers vary from person to person. For some, it might be stress or anxiety, for others, it could be a place, a group of friends, or even a time of day. Social events, celebrations, or even certain emotions can act as triggers. It's essential to recognize that triggers are not just external; they can be internal, rooted in our emotions and thoughts.

Everyone's journey with alcoholism is unique, and so are their triggers. It's vital to create a personalized list, a roadmap of potential pitfalls. This list becomes a tool, a guide to navigate the treacherous waters of recovery.

Dialectical Behavior Therapy (DBT) offers a fresh perspective on managing triggers. Instead of merely avoiding them, DBT equips individuals with the skills to face them head-on.

Mindfulness is the art of being present. By practicing mindfulness, one can become acutely aware of their surroundings, emotions, and thoughts. This heightened awareness acts as an early warning system, signaling the approach of a potential trigger.

DBT offers a plethora of techniques to divert the mind from the trigger, from deep breathing exercises to visualization techniques. The goal is not to suppress the urge but to redirect it, to channel it into a more positive outlet.

Like any skill, recognizing triggers requires practice. Through various exercises, from journaling to role-playing, one can hone this skill, making it second nature.

Resilience is the armor against triggers, the shield that guards against relapse.

Life is filled with distressing situations, but with DBT, one learns to tolerate distress without resorting to alcohol. It's about enduring the storm, knowing that clear skies await.

Sometimes, despite all precautions, one might face a trigger head-on. In such situations, having a strategy, a plan of action, can make all the difference. Whether it's calling a friend, practicing deep breathing, or engaging in a distraction activity, these immediate response strategies can be lifesavers.

Building resilience is an ongoing process. By regularly reflecting on one's experiences, feelings, and reactions, one can gain insights, strengthening their resilience further.

To truly grasp the concept of triggers, we must venture into the realm of neuroscience. Our brain, a marvel of nature, is wired in intricate ways, and its pathways play a pivotal role in addiction and recovery.

When an individual consumes alcohol, especially in excessive amounts over time, the brain releases dopamine, a neurotransmitter associated with pleasure and reward. Over time, the brain starts associating certain stimuli with this dopamine release. These stimuli, or triggers, can be anything: a place, a song, a scent, or even an emotion. When encountered, these triggers create a powerful urge to drink, seeking that dopamine rush.

But here's the silver lining. Just as our brain can be conditioned to associate stimuli with alcohol, it can also be retrained. This is where DBT comes into play. Through mindfulness and other DBT techniques, individuals can rewire their brain, creating new associations, and breaking the cycle of addiction.

Dialectical Behavior Therapy, or DBT, is not just another therapy. It's a lifeline for many on the path of recovery. Originally developed to treat borderline personality disorder, its principles have shown remarkable efficacy in treating a range of conditions, including alcoholism.

Traditional therapies often focus on the 'why' – why did the addiction start, why does one continue to drink, and so on. While understanding the root cause is essential, it's often not enough. DBT, on the other hand, emphasizes the 'how'. How can one recognize triggers? How can one manage cravings? How can one build a life worth living without alcohol? It's a more proactive, hands-on approach, equipping individuals with practical skills for real-world challenges.

At its core, DBT combines the principles of cognitive-behavioral therapy with mindfulness practices derived from Buddhist meditative traditions. This fusion addresses both the emotional and behavioral aspects of addiction. By teaching individuals to be present, to be aware of their emotions, thoughts, and surroundings, DBT helps in early recognition of triggers. And by imparting skills like distress tolerance and emotional regulation, it ensures that even when faced with a trigger, the individual has the tools to navigate it.

While the core principles of DBT remain constant, its application for alcoholism has nuances. It's not just about avoiding alcohol; it's about building a life where alcohol becomes irrelevant. It's about finding joy in sobriety, about mending relationships strained by addiction, and about rediscovering oneself.

Mindfulness, a cornerstone of DBT, is more than just a buzzword. It's a transformative practice that has its roots in ancient meditative traditions. But what does it mean to be mindful, especially in the context of alcohol recovery?

Being mindful means being fully present, being acutely aware of one's emotions, thoughts, and surroundings without judgment. It's about observing oneself, almost like an outsider, and recognizing patterns. In the realm of alcohol recovery, this heightened self-awareness is invaluable.

Imagine walking into a room and feeling a sudden urge to drink. Instead of succumbing to the urge or chastising oneself for feeling it, mindfulness teaches us to pause and observe. What triggered this urge? Was it the ambiance, a particular scent, a song playing in the background, or perhaps a memory associated with the place? By being mindful, one can identify these triggers, understand them, and eventually, neutralize their power.

Recognizing triggers is just one part of the equation. The next step, and often the more challenging one, is managing the response to these triggers. This is where DBT shines, offering a plethora of techniques tailored for this very purpose.

One such technique is the STOP skill. STOP stands for:

- (S)top: When faced with a trigger, pause. Do not react impulsively.

- (T)ake a step back: Disengage from the situation, even if it's just mentally. Create a buffer.

- (O)bserve: What are you feeling? What's the intensity of the urge? Is there an underlying emotion driving it?

- (P)roceed mindfully: Armed with this awareness, make a conscious choice. It could be to leave the situation, engage in a distraction, or use another DBT skill.

Another powerful technique is the TIPP skill, designed to change one's body chemistry and reduce emotional arousal. It involves:

- (T)emperature: Splashing cold water on the face or holding a cold pack can calm overwhelming emotions.

- (I)ntense exercise: A short burst of physical activity can help in burning off the distressing emotions.

- (P)aced breathing: Slow, deep breaths can have a calming effect.

- (P)aired muscle relaxation: Tensing and then relaxing muscle groups can help in grounding oneself.

While understanding these techniques is essential, the real magic happens when one practices them. Here are a few exercises tailored for trigger recognition:

1. Mindful Journaling: Every evening, spend a few minutes reflecting on the day. Were there moments when you felt the urge to drink? What triggered it? How did you respond? Over time, this journal can offer valuable insights into your unique triggers and patterns.

2. Mindful Meditation: Dedicate a few minutes each day to sit in silence, focusing on your breath. If your mind wanders, gently bring it back. This simple practice can enhance self-awareness and make trigger recognition almost second nature.

3. Role-playing: With a trusted friend or therapist, recreate scenarios where you've previously faced triggers. Practice using DBT skills in these simulated settings. This not only reinforces the skills but also boosts confidence in handling real-life situations.

Resilience is not just the ability to bounce back from setbacks; it's the capacity to grow and thrive in the face of challenges. In the context of alcohol recovery, resilience means not just avoiding relapse but building a life of purpose, joy, and fulfillment.

Increasing distress tolerance is a significant aspect of this. Life will always have its ups and downs, but with heightened distress tolerance, one can navigate these without resorting to alcohol. DBT offers a range of skills for this, from radical acceptance to self-soothing techniques.

Strategies for immediate trigger response are equally crucial. It's about having an arsenal of tools at one's disposal and knowing instinctively which one to use when faced with a trigger. Over time, with practice, these responses become ingrained, almost automatic.

Lastly, the role of self-awareness and reflection cannot be overstated. By regularly reflecting on one's journey, celebrating the victories, learning from the setbacks, and continuously realigning with one's goals, one can ensure that the path of recovery is not just about avoiding alcohol but about holistic personal growth.

The journey through understanding the intricate dance between DBT and alcoholism is both enlightening and empowering. As we reflect on the chapter, several pivotal insights emerge that can serve as guiding lights on the path to recovery.

1. The Power of Mindfulness: At the heart of DBT lies mindfulness, a practice that transcends mere awareness. It's about being present, observing without judgment, and understanding oneself deeply. In the context of alcoholism, mindfulness becomes an invaluable tool. It allows one to recognize triggers, understand their roots, and respond to them consciously rather than reactively. By cultivating a mindful approach, one can navigate the treacherous waters of recovery with greater clarity and purpose.

2. DBT's Multifaceted Approach to Triggers: Recognizing triggers is just the beginning. DBT offers a rich tapestry of techniques to manage and mitigate the power of these triggers. From the STOP skill, which emphasizes pausing and observing, to the TIPP skill, which focuses on physiological interventions, DBT provides a comprehensive toolkit. These tools, when applied consistently, can transform one's relationship with triggers, making them less daunting and more manageable.

3. The Emphasis on Practice: Knowledge, while powerful, is only the first step. The real transformation occurs when one puts this knowledge into practice. Through exercises like mindful journaling, meditation, and role-playing, one can internalize the principles of DBT. Over time, these practices not only enhance trigger recognition but also bolster confidence in managing them.

4. Building Resilience: Recovery is not just about avoiding relapse; it's about building a life of meaning, purpose, and joy. DBT places a

strong emphasis on building resilience, which is the ability to navigate life's challenges with grace and poise. By increasing distress tolerance and cultivating strategies for immediate trigger response, one can build a robust foundation for long-term recovery.

5. The Role of Reflection: The journey of recovery is filled with peaks and valleys. Regular reflection allows one to celebrate the victories, learn from the setbacks, and realign with one's goals. It ensures that the path of recovery is not just reactive but proactive, driven by a clear vision and purpose.

6. Holistic Personal Growth: DBT's approach to alcohol recovery is holistic. It's not just about abstaining from alcohol but about personal growth, improving interpersonal relationships, and building a life of fulfillment. By integrating the principles of DBT, one can embark on a journey that is as much about self-discovery as it is about recovery.

In essence, this chapter underscores the transformative power of DBT in the realm of alcohol recovery. It paints a picture of hope, empowerment, and transformation, emphasizing that with the right tools and mindset, recovery is not just possible but achievable.

As we close this enlightening chapter on the essence of DBT and its profound implications in alcohol recovery, it's essential to remember that understanding is just the beginning. The next chapter will delve deeper, exploring the practical applications of these principles. We'll embark on a journey that will not only illuminate the path of recovery but also provide actionable steps to walk it with confidence and purpose. Join us as we continue to unravel the intricacies of DBT and its transformative potential.

# Chapter Three

---

# Emotional Regulation in Depth

The room was dimly lit, with the faint hum of a ceiling fan echoing in the background. Sarah sat on her couch, her hands trembling. The weight of the world seemed to press down on her shoulders. Memories of past failures, regrets, and the haunting feeling of inadequacy consumed her. She felt overwhelmed, trapped in a whirlwind of emotions she couldn't control. Before she knew it, she found herself reaching for the bottle she had sworn off months ago. The emotional storm had led her back to the very thing she was trying to escape.

Emotions, when left unchecked, can become powerful drivers of our actions, leading us down paths we later regret. This chapter delves deep into the realm of emotional dysregulation, its ties to addiction, and how DBT offers tools and techniques to navigate this tumultuous landscape. We'll explore the intricate dance between emotions and relapse, and how one can harness the power of DBT to maintain emotional equilibrium.

Emotional dysregulation, at its core, is the inability to manage intense emotions effectively. It's like being on a roller coaster without a safety harness, where every twist and turn threatens to throw you off balance. For many, these emotional upheavals are not just occasional occurrences but a daily struggle.

But what causes this turbulence? Several factors come into play. From biological predispositions, traumatic experiences, to environmental stressors, the roots of emotional dysregulation can be multifaceted. It's essential to understand that it's not just about "overreacting." It's a complex interplay of internal and external factors that disrupt one's emotional equilibrium.

In the realm of addiction, especially alcoholism, emotional dysregulation plays a pivotal role. The overwhelming emotions often become triggers, pushing individuals towards substances as a means of escape. It's a vicious cycle. The very thing one uses to cope exacerbates the problem, leading to feelings of guilt, shame, and further emotional turmoil.

Moreover, there's a profound connection between emotional dysregulation and mental health. Conditions like Borderline Personality Disorder, PTSD, and even depression have emotional dysregulation as a hallmark symptom. Recognizing this connection is crucial as it underscores the importance of addressing emotional dysregulation in the broader context of mental well-being.

Recognizing one's emotional patterns is the first step towards healing. It's about understanding the triggers, the emotional responses, and the subsequent actions. DBT offers a rich array of techniques to navigate this process. Imagine being in the eye of a storm. Around you, emotions rage, but with DBT, you can find that calm center, that place of clarity and control.

One of the foundational exercises in DBT is mindfulness meditation. It's not just about sitting in silence but actively observing one's emotions without judgment. It's about understanding the ebb and flow of feelings, recognizing them as transient, and not getting swept away.

But what happens when emotions become too overwhelming? DBT offers strategies for de-escalation. Techniques like deep breathing, grounding exercises, and even sensory diversions can help divert the emotional tide, giving one a momentary respite to regroup and respond rather than react.

While techniques and strategies are vital, consistency is the key to lasting change. Emotional regulation is not a destination but a journey, one that requires daily practice and reflection. Journaling, for instance, can be a powerful tool. It's a space to reflect, to understand patterns, and to celebrate progress.

Moreover, the role of consistency cannot be overstated. Just like a muscle, emotional regulation requires regular exercise. Whether it's daily mindfulness practice, regular check-ins with one's emotional state, or even seeking support when needed, maintaining emotional balance is an ongoing process.

The intricate tapestry of our emotions is woven with threads of various experiences, memories, and inherent predispositions. While it's easy to attribute emotional upheavals solely to external triggers or specific events, the underlying mental health landscape plays a significant role in shaping these responses.

Consider, for a moment, a serene lake. On the surface, it's calm, reflecting the sky and trees. But beneath, there might be currents, unseen creatures, and various depths. Similarly, our emotional responses, which appear on the surface, are influenced by underlying mental health conditions, past traumas, and inherent predispositions.

For instance, someone with a history of trauma might experience heightened emotional responses to seemingly benign triggers. A sudden loud noise or an unexpected touch might evoke intense feelings of fear or anger. This isn't merely an "overreaction" but a deeply ingrained protective response developed over time.

Similarly, conditions like Borderline Personality Disorder (BPD) are characterized by intense emotional responses and a pattern of unstable relationships. For someone with BPD, the fear of abandonment might trigger intense emotions, leading to behaviors that, from an external perspective, might seem disproportionate.

Dialectical Behavior Therapy (DBT) recognizes the profound impact of these underlying conditions and offers tools tailored to address them. It's not a one-size-fits-all approach but a nuanced, individualized strategy that takes into account the person's unique mental health landscape.

Mindfulness, a core component of DBT, is more than a buzzword. It's a practice that encourages individuals to stay present, to observe their emotions without judgment, and to respond rather than react. For someone with a history of trauma, mindfulness can offer a momentary pause, a space to breathe, and an opportunity to choose a different response.

Similarly, DBT emphasizes the importance of emotional validation. It's about recognizing and affirming one's feelings, understanding that they are real and valid, even if they seem intense or disproportionate. This validation can be profoundly healing, especially for those who've often been told that they're "too sensitive" or "overreacting."

While understanding and validation are crucial, they are but the first steps on the journey of emotional regulation. The path forward requires consistent practice, reflection, and, at times, guidance.

Imagine learning to play a musical instrument. The initial notes might sound discordant, but with practice, they transform into a melody. Similarly, the journey of emotional regulation is filled with highs and lows, moments of discord, and harmony.

Journaling, as mentioned earlier, can be a powerful ally in this journey. It offers a space to reflect, to understand patterns, and to celebrate progress. Moreover, it provides a tangible record of one's journey, a testament to the challenges overcome and the growth achieved.

Furthermore, the importance of seeking support, whether through therapy, support groups, or trusted confidants, cannot be overstated. Emotional regulation, especially in the context of addiction recovery, is not a solitary journey. It's a path best walked with support, guidance, and, most importantly, hope.

The journey of recovery, especially from alcoholism, is akin to navigating a labyrinth. There are twists and turns, dead ends, and moments of clarity. The walls of this maze are often built from past traumas, emotional upheavals, societal judgments, and deeply ingrained habits. But what if there was a map? A guide that, while not eliminating the challenges, provides a clearer path forward? Dialectical Behavior Therapy (DBT) offers just that.

At its core, DBT is not merely a set of techniques or exercises. It's a philosophy, a way of viewing oneself, the world, and the intricate dance of emotions and behaviors. Founded by Marsha Linehan, DBT was initially developed to address the unique challenges faced by individuals with Borderline Personality Disorder. However, its principles, deeply rooted in mindfulness, acceptance, and change, found resonance in various other areas, including addiction recovery.

For someone grappling with alcoholism, the allure of the bottle isn't just about the physical craving. It's often an escape, a momentary relief from the tumultuous storm of emotions. Feelings of guilt, shame, anger, or sadness can become overwhelming, and in that moment of intense vulnerability, alcohol promises a refuge. But, as many realize, it's a false sanctuary, one that often exacerbates the emotional turmoil.

One of the foundational pillars of DBT is mindfulness. Now, this isn't about sitting cross-legged and chanting (unless that's what resonates with you). It's about being present, deeply and wholly, in the current moment. For someone in the throes of emotional dysregulation, this might seem like a Herculean task. The past and the future often hold the mind hostage, with memories of past mistakes or anxieties about future relapses.

But mindfulness offers a pause button. A moment to breathe, to observe without judgment. It's like being in the eye of the storm, where, for a brief moment, everything is calm. In this space, there's clarity, an opportunity to choose a response rather than being swept away in a reactive whirlwind.

DBT offers various techniques for emotional grounding. Imagine standing on the deck of a ship amidst a storm. The waves are tumultuous, threatening to sweep you away. But then you find an anchor, something to hold onto, to ground yourself. Emotional grounding techniques serve as this anchor.

One such technique is the "5-4-3-2-1" sensory awareness exercise. When emotions become overwhelming, take a moment to identify:

- Five things you can see

- Four you can touch

- Three you can hear

- Two you can smell

- One you can taste

This simple exercise, rooted in the present moment, can offer a brief respite, a chance to recalibrate.

Understanding and implementing DBT techniques is a journey, not a destination. It requires practice, patience, and, most importantly, self-compassion. There will be moments of relapse, moments of doubt, but each step, each moment of mindfulness, each instance of emotional grounding, is a step forward.

Emotional dysregulation, at its core, is an inability to manage intense emotions effectively. It's like trying to hold back a tidal wave with a mere sandbag. The pressure builds, and without the right tools or understanding, a breach is inevitable. For many, this breach manifests as a return to the bottle, seeking solace in its numbing embrace.

To truly grasp the concept of emotional dysregulation, one must first dive into its origins. For some, it's rooted in past traumas, experiences that have left deep emotional scars. For others, it might be a result of chronic stress, societal pressures, or even underlying mental health conditions. The common thread, however, is the overwhelming nature of these emotions. It's not just feeling sad; it's a profound despair. It's not mere worry; it's paralyzing anxiety.

Marsha Linehan, the founder of DBT, recognized the profound impact of emotional dysregulation on one's life. She saw individuals, deeply suffering, caught in a cycle of self-destructive behaviors, not out of choice, but out of a desperate need for relief. Her contribution to the field of psychology, and more specifically to the realm of addiction recovery, is monumental. She didn't just provide a set of techniques; she offered a lifeline, a beacon of hope.

While DBT was not initially designed for addiction recovery, its principles found a natural fit. The core tenets of mindfulness, distress tolerance, emotional regulation, and interpersonal effectiveness provided the tools individuals needed to navigate the stormy seas of recovery.

Imagine being trapped in a room with an ever-growing balloon. That balloon represents the mounting emotions, the pressures, the triggers. Without an outlet, without a way to release some of that pressure, an explosion is inevitable. DBT provides the tools to slowly and methodically release that pressure, ensuring the balloon never reaches its breaking point.

Consider the story of Alex, a 35-year-old who had battled alcoholism for over a decade. On the surface, Alex had it all – a loving family, a successful career, and a vibrant social life. But beneath that veneer lay a tumultuous emotional landscape. Every setback, every perceived slight, every stressor was a potential trigger. Alex described it as "walking on a tightrope over a chasm of despair."

When Alex was introduced to DBT, it wasn't a magical panacea. The first few sessions were challenging, even confrontational. But as Alex delved deeper into the principles of mindfulness and emotional regulation, a transformation began. Alex learned to recognize the early signs of emotional upheaval, to pause and reflect rather than react. Over time, the tightrope became a bridge, and the chasm less daunting.

Emotional dysregulation isn't merely about experiencing intense emotions; it's about the overwhelming struggle to manage them. It's akin to trying to contain a tempest in a teapot. The pressure, the intensity, and the sheer force of these emotions can lead individuals down paths they never intended to tread. For many, especially those battling alcoholism, it becomes a desperate attempt to find solace, even if that solace is momentarily found at the bottom of a bottle.

Every individual's journey with emotional dysregulation is unique, shaped by past traumas, societal pressures, chronic stress, or underlying mental health conditions. It's essential to recognize that these aren't fleeting feelings but profound emotional states. It's not about feeling momentarily down; it's about experiencing a depth of despair that seems endless. It's not about a passing worry; it's about an anxiety that feels all-consuming.

Marsha Linehan didn't just introduce a therapy; she provided a lifeline. Recognizing the profound suffering of individuals trapped in cycles of self-destructive behaviors, she offered hope. Her approach, Dialectical Behavior Therapy (DBT), wasn't just a set of techniques but a holistic approach to managing and understanding emotions. It was about offering individuals the tools they needed to navigate their emotional landscapes effectively.

DBT, though not initially designed for addiction recovery, seamlessly integrated into it. Its core principles, ranging from mindfulness to emotional regulation, provided the much-needed tools for those in recovery. It was about recognizing triggers, understanding emotional responses, and equipping individuals with strategies to manage them. It wasn't about avoiding emotions but understanding and navigating them.

Stories like Alex's aren't unique but are a testament to the transformative power of DBT. It's about individuals, once trapped in their emotional maelstroms, finding clarity and purpose. It's about recognizing triggers, understanding emotional patterns, and equipping oneself with the tools to navigate them. It's about turning the tightrope of recovery into a bridge of hope.

Recovery, as with any profound journey, is filled with its share of challenges and triumphs. But with tools like DBT, the path becomes clearer, the challenges more manageable, and the triumphs more profound. It's about understanding that recovery isn't a destination but a journey, and with every step taken, no matter how small, progress is made.

As we draw this chapter to a close, it's essential to pause and reflect on the transformative power of DBT, especially in the realm of alcoholism. We've delved deep into the intricacies of emotional dysregulation, the pioneering work of Marsha Linehan, and the profound impact of DBT techniques in the recovery journey. But this is just the beginning. The world of recovery is vast, with many facets and layers waiting to be explored. Our next chapter promises to take you deeper into this journey, unraveling more insights and tools that can be your guiding light. As we transition, let's carry forward the knowledge we've gained, using it as a foundation to build upon, ensuring that every step we take is informed, purposeful, and geared towards a brighter, more empowered future.

# Chapter Four

---

# Mindfulness and Present Living

H ave you ever found yourself lost in a moment, so engrossed in the present that the past and future seemed to blur? What if that wasn't just a fleeting experience but a way of life?

In this chapter, we'll embark on a journey through the serene landscapes of mindfulness. From its ancient roots to its modern applications, we'll delve into how mindfulness has become an integral part of Dialectical Behavior Therapy (DBT) and its profound impact on recovery from alcoholism.

Mindfulness, though a buzzword in today's wellness circles, is not a new concept. Its roots trace back thousands of years, deeply embedded in the teachings of Buddhism. Ancient monks practiced mindfulness as a path to enlightenment, a way to truly understand the self and the world. But what was once a spiritual practice has now found its way into the modern world, not as a religious doctrine, but as a therapeutic tool.

The essence of mindfulness lies in its simplicity: being present. It's about immersing oneself in the current moment, observing without judgment. This might sound easy, but in a world filled with distractions, it's a profound challenge. Yet, the beauty of mindfulness is that it's not about achieving a state of eternal calm but about recognizing and accepting our thoughts and emotions, no matter how tumultuous.

A common misconception is equating mindfulness with meditation. While they share similarities, they are distinct practices. Meditation is a structured practice, often involving specific postures, breathing techniques, and sometimes mantras. It's about setting aside dedicated time to focus inward. Mindfulness, on the other hand, is a way of life. It's about being present in every moment, whether you're meditating, walking, eating, or even engaged in a conversation.

Imagine walking in a forest. Meditation would be like finding a serene spot, sitting down, closing your eyes, and focusing on your breath or the sounds around you. Mindfulness would be feeling the crunch of leaves underfoot, noticing the play of sunlight through the trees, feeling the breeze on your skin, and hearing the distant call of birds. Both practices offer a path to inner peace, but they guide you there differently.

Dialectical Behavior Therapy, pioneered by Marsha Linehan, recognized the transformative power of mindfulness. In the context of DBT, mindfulness isn't just about being present; it's about learning to regulate emotions, tolerate distress, and improve interpersonal relationships. It's a tool, a skill, and a way of life.

DBT offers a range of techniques and exercises to cultivate mindfulness. From "Wise Mind" exercises that help individuals find the balance between emotional and rational thinking to "Observation and Description" exercises that teach the art of observing without judgment and describing without interpretation. These techniques are not just theoretical constructs but practical tools, designed to be integrated into daily life.

For someone battling alcoholism, these exercises become even more crucial. The journey of recovery is fraught with challenges, from confronting past traumas to dealing with cravings. Mindfulness, in this context, becomes a beacon, guiding individuals away from impulsive decisions and towards thoughtful reflection.

The benefits of mindfulness in recovery are manifold. At its core, mindfulness teaches self-awareness. For someone in recovery, this means recognizing triggers, understanding emotional responses, and making informed choices. It's about breaking the cycle of impulsivity that often leads to relapse.

Moreover, mindfulness enhances distress tolerance. Cravings, memories, and emotions can be overwhelming, but mindfulness offers a way to navigate this storm. It teaches individuals to sit with their discomfort, observe it, and let it pass without acting on it.

Mindfulness plays a pivotal role in relapse prevention. By fostering self-awareness and distress tolerance, it equips individuals with the tools they need to face challenges head-on, reducing the risk of relapse.

Mindfulness isn't just a tool for those in recovery from alcoholism; its benefits extend to the broader realm of mental health. In a world that's increasingly fast-paced, where stressors lurk around every corner, mental well-being often takes a back seat. Here, mindfulness emerges as a beacon of hope.

When we talk about mental health, we're referring to a spectrum. On one end, there are diagnosed conditions like depression, anxiety, and bipolar disorder. On the other, there's the day-to-day stress, anxiety, and emotional turbulence that many of us experience. Mindfulness, with its emphasis on living in the present, offers relief across this spectrum.

Imagine the mind as a turbulent sea. The waves represent our thoughts, emotions, and reactions. Sometimes these waves are gentle, lapping at the shores, and at other times, they're tumultuous, threatening to engulf everything in their path. Mindfulness teaches us to observe these waves from the shore, without getting swept away. It's about recognizing that while we can't control the sea, we can choose our response to it.

For someone with a diagnosed mental health condition, this can be transformative. Traditional therapies often focus on understanding the 'why' – why do I feel this way? Why did I react like that? Mindfulness shifts the focus to the 'what' – what am I feeling right now? What can I do about it? This shift, subtle yet profound, can make all the difference.

Dialectical Behavior Therapy (DBT) and mindfulness share a deep, symbiotic relationship. While DBT integrates mindfulness as one of its core components, mindfulness, in turn, draws strength from the structured approach of DBT.

DBT, with its emphasis on balancing acceptance and change, finds a natural ally in mindfulness. Mindfulness teaches acceptance – of the self, of the present moment, of our thoughts and emotions. But it also empowers change. By fostering self-awareness, it equips individuals with the insights they need to make informed choices, to break free from patterns that no longer serve them.

In the context of alcohol recovery, this relationship becomes even more crucial. Alcoholism isn't just about the physical addiction; it's deeply intertwined with emotional pain, trauma, and patterns of behavior. DBT, with its structured approach, offers a roadmap to recovery. Mindfulness, with its emphasis on living in the present, illuminates this roadmap, ensuring that individuals don't lose their way.

Like any other skill, mindfulness requires practice. It's not a switch that you can turn on and off; it's a muscle that you need to flex regularly. And just like any other muscle, the more you exercise it, the stronger it becomes.

Consistency in mindfulness practice is crucial. It's not about setting aside hours every day; it's about integrating it into the fabric of daily life. It's about choosing to be present, whether you're brushing your teeth, eating a meal, or taking a walk. It's about recognizing that every moment offers an opportunity to practice mindfulness.

For someone in recovery, this consistency can be a lifeline. The journey of recovery is filled with ups and downs. There will be moments of clarity and moments of doubt, moments of strength, and moments of weakness. Consistent mindfulness practice offers a grounding force, a touchstone that individuals can return to, no matter where they are on their journey.

The journey of recovery, as we've delved into, is not just about abstaining from alcohol. It's a transformative process, a reclamation of self, and at its heart lies the power of mindfulness. Here are the pivotal takeaways from our exploration:

1. The Antidote to Impulsiveness: At the core of addiction lies impulsiveness, the immediate need that often blindsides long-term consequences. Mindfulness, with its emphasis on the present moment, acts as a buffer. It doesn't suppress the urge but allows for understanding and recognition. By being present, the immediacy of the impulse diminishes, granting the individual the space to choose a response rather than react out of habit.

2. Journey to Self-awareness: Mindfulness is a mirror, reflecting not just our actions but our motivations, desires, and fears. For someone in recovery, this self-awareness is a beacon. It's about understanding the 'why' behind the addiction, recognizing patterns, and charting a new path forward. Through mindfulness, one embarks on a journey of self-discovery, understanding both strengths and weaknesses.

3. Relapse as a Stepping Stone: Relapse, while challenging, is a part of many individuals' recovery journey. Instead of viewing it as a setback, through the lens of mindfulness, it becomes a stepping stone, an opportunity for growth and understanding. Mindfulness plays a pivotal role in relapse prevention by building resilience and equipping individuals with the tools to navigate recovery's challenges.

4. The Lifelong Commitment: Both mindfulness and recovery are processes, not end goals. They are intertwined journeys of growth, understanding, and transformation. The beauty of mindfulness is its simplicity and its promise of a life lived in the present, with purpose, meaning, and joy.

5. The Role of DBT: While this chapter focused on mindfulness, it's essential to recognize its place within the broader framework of Dialectical Behavior Therapy (DBT). Mindfulness is but one facet of DBT, and its true potential is realized when combined with other techniques and strategies, something we'll delve deeper into in subsequent chapters.

In essence, the journey of recovery, when combined with the power of mindfulness, becomes not just about abstaining from alcohol but about reclaiming one's life. It's about living each moment with purpose, understanding oneself, and charting a path forward filled with hope, promise, and joy.

As the curtains draw on this chapter, we find ourselves on the cusp of a broader horizon. The essence of mindfulness, its roots, and its profound impact on recovery have been our focus. But as with any intricate tapestry, there are more threads to unravel. The next chapter beckons us to delve deeper into the vast realm of Dialectical Behavior Therapy. While mindfulness is a shining gem in the crown of DBT, there are other facets, equally radiant and essential, waiting to be explored. We'll journey through the corridors of DBT, understanding its origins, its principles, and its unparalleled role in the world of recovery. As we transition, let's carry with us the lessons of mindfulness, for they will be the guiding light, illuminating the path as we delve deeper into the therapeutic wonders of DBT. The next chapter is not just a continuation; it's a deepening, an expansion, and a promise of a more profound understanding. So, with anticipation in our hearts and curiosity as our compass, let's step forward into this enlightening journey.

# Chapter Five

---

# Mending Relationships and Interpersonal Effectiveness

T he room was filled with the deafening silence of unsaid words. Sarah looked across the table, trying to find the man she once knew in the eyes of the stranger before her. Alcohol had not just taken away his sobriety; it had chipped away at the very foundation of their relationship.

Relationships are the bedrock of our existence. They provide support, love, and a sense of belonging. However, the corrosive nature of alcoholism can erode these bonds, leaving behind pain and mistrust. In this chapter, we will delve deep into the impact of alcoholism on relationships, exploring personal narratives and understanding the broader implications. More importantly, we will discover how Dialectical Behavior Therapy (DBT) can act as a bridge, mending broken ties and fostering healthier connections.

Alcoholism is not a solitary disease. It casts a wide net, ensnaring not just the individual but everyone around them. Relationships, whether familial, romantic, or platonic, bear the brunt of this affliction. The joyous moments are overshadowed by unpredictability, broken promises, and emotional withdrawal. Trust, once the cornerstone of these bonds, often becomes the first casualty.

To truly understand the impact, we turn to stories. James, a recovering alcoholic, shares his journey of pushing away his loved ones, blinded by his addiction. On the other hand, we hear from Emily, a daughter who watched her father transform under the influence, yearning for the moments of clarity when he remembered her name. These narratives, though heart-wrenching, also carry a message of hope and resilience.

It's not just the immediate relationships that suffer. The ripple effect of alcoholism touches friends, colleagues, and even acquaintances. The unpredictability associated with alcoholism means that social gatherings become a source of anxiety. Family members often find themselves walking on eggshells, anticipating the next outburst or breakdown.

Enter Dialectical Behavior Therapy. DBT, with its emphasis on mindfulness, emotional regulation, and interpersonal effectiveness, offers a ray of hope. Through various strategies, it equips individuals with the tools to communicate effectively, understand the perspectives of others, and most importantly, rebuild trust.

Communication is the lifeline of any relationship. DBT emphasizes the importance of being present during interactions, actively listening, and expressing oneself clearly. Techniques such as "DEAR MAN" provide a structured approach to making requests or asserting oneself, ensuring that the communication is effective and respectful.

Empathy plays a crucial role in mending relationships. DBT exercises focus on understanding and validating the emotions of others. By putting oneself in their shoes, it becomes easier to grasp their perspective, paving the way for mutual understanding.

Recovery is not a destination but a journey. Similarly, sustaining healthy relationships requires continuous effort. Regular reflection, open communication, and the application of DBT techniques ensure that relationships remain strong, even in the face of challenges.

Conflicts are inevitable in any relationship. However, with the tools provided by DBT, individuals can navigate these conflicts without resorting to old patterns. By recognizing triggers, employing distress tolerance techniques, and communicating effectively, conflicts can be resolved in a healthy manner.

In the realm of relationships marred by alcoholism, self-awareness emerges as a beacon of hope. It's not just about recognizing one's patterns of behavior but delving deeper into understanding the 'why' behind them. Why did a particular comment trigger an outburst? Why does a specific memory lead to feelings of guilt? These are the questions that, when answered, pave the way for genuine healing.

Self-awareness, as promoted by DBT, is not a mere introspective exercise. It's a journey of understanding oneself in relation to others. It's about recognizing the impact of one's actions on those around them. For someone recovering from alcoholism, this could mean understanding the pain their addiction has caused their loved ones. For a partner or family member, it might be about realizing the ways they've perhaps enabled the behavior or the protective walls they've built over time.

One of the most potent tools for enhancing self-awareness is journaling. The act of putting pen to paper, or fingers to keys in today's digital age, allows for a stream of consciousness to flow. It's an unfiltered, raw, and often enlightening experience. Over time, patterns emerge from these journal entries. Patterns of behavior, of thought processes, and of triggers.

For someone in recovery, a journal can serve as both a confidante and a record of progress. It can be a place to vent, to express guilt, remorse, hope, and joy. But more than that, it can be a tool for reflection. Reading back on entries can offer insights into how far one has come, the challenges they've overcome, and the hurdles yet to be tackled.

Healing, especially in relationships scarred by addiction, is not an overnight process. It's a journey, often filled with two steps forward and one step back. But the key lies in consistency. Consistency in effort, in communication, and in applying the tools and techniques learned through DBT.

Every day presents a new opportunity. An opportunity to mend, to build, and to grow. And every effort, no matter how small, contributes to the larger goal of healing. It's like building a mosaic, piece by piece, with each piece representing an effort, an apology, a moment of understanding, or a gesture of love.

Vulnerability, often misconstrued as a sign of weakness, is in fact a testament to courage. In the context of relationships affected by alcoholism, embracing vulnerability can be the bridge to genuine connection and understanding. It's about laying bare one's fears, regrets, and hopes, allowing for a space of mutual empathy.

Imagine standing at the edge of a precipice, the wind howling around, and taking that leap, not knowing if you'll fly or fall. That's vulnerability. And in that leap, in that moment of uncertainty, lies the potential for profound connection. For someone recovering from alcoholism, this could mean sharing their deepest fears about relapse or their guilt over past actions. For a loved one, it might be about expressing the pain of feeling neglected or the fear of losing the person they care about to addiction.

While expressing oneself is a significant part of the healing process, so is listening. Active listening, to be precise. It's not just about hearing the words but understanding the emotions and sentiments behind them. It's about being present, fully and completely, offering a safe space for the other person to express themselves.

Imagine a scenario where a recovering individual shares their fear of relapse. Active listening would involve not just hearing that fear but understanding the myriad emotions tied to it – the guilt, the pressure, the desire to change. It's about offering validation, comfort, and, most importantly, a non-judgmental ear.

Trust, once broken, is challenging to rebuild. But it's not impossible. In relationships marred by alcoholism, trust is often one of the biggest casualties. But with effort, understanding, and time, it can be restored.

The key lies in consistency and transparency. It's about showing up, every day, making an effort, being honest, and taking responsibility. For a recovering individual, this could mean being open about their struggles, seeking help when needed, and honoring their commitments. For a loved one, it might involve setting boundaries, expressing their needs, and offering support without enabling.

Life is replete with stories of second chances, of phoenixes rising from the ashes, of rainbows after storms. Relationships, even those strained by the weight of addiction, are no different. With effort, understanding, and love, they can find a new lease on life.

One of the most profound revelations from our exploration is the transformative power of vulnerability. In a world where strength is often equated with stoicism, the act of opening oneself up, of revealing one's fears and hopes, stands as a testament to true courage. Vulnerability is not about weakness; it's about forging deeper connections, understanding, and mutual empathy. It's the bridge that spans the chasm of misunderstandings and hurt, especially in relationships strained by alcoholism.

Communication isn't just about speaking; it's equally about listening. But not just any listening - active listening. This involves immersing oneself fully in the moment, understanding the emotions behind the words, and offering a safe, non-judgmental space for the other person. It's a two-way street where both parties feel seen, heard, and valued. In the context of relationships affected by alcoholism, active listening can be the salve that soothes old wounds and paves the way for genuine understanding.

Trust, once shattered, demands time, patience, and consistent effort to rebuild. It's a delicate dance of taking responsibility, being transparent, and showing up every day. For relationships marred by alcoholism, restoring trust is paramount. It's about the recovering individual being open about their journey, the challenges, the triumphs, and the setbacks. It's also about loved ones setting boundaries, expressing their needs, and offering support without falling into the trap of enabling.

Life, in its infinite wisdom, often offers second chances. Relationships, even those strained to breaking point by addiction, can find renewal and hope. It's a testament to the indomitable human spirit, the capacity to forgive, to grow, and to love again. Every day presents a new opportunity, a fresh slate, and the promise of a brighter tomorrow.

The techniques and strategies offered by Dialectical Behavior Therapy (DBT) are invaluable tools in this journey of healing. From promoting active listening to fostering emotional regulation, DBT provides a roadmap for individuals and their loved ones to navigate the choppy waters of addiction and find their way back to each other.

As we conclude this enlightening chapter on the profound impact of alcoholism on relationships and the beacon of hope that DBT provides, we find ourselves on the cusp of yet another transformative exploration. The forthcoming chapter will guide us deeper into the realm of alcohol recovery using DBT, shedding light on its intricate facets and revealing its profound implications in the context of addiction and recovery. With the knowledge and insights we've accumulated thus far, we are better equipped to navigate the complexities ahead, understanding the nuances and appreciating the subtleties. Let's journey forward, hand in hand, as we continue to unravel the mysteries of the human psyche, addiction, and the path to healing.

# Chapter Six

---

# Mastering Distress Tolerance

D id you know that a significant number of relapses in alcoholism are triggered not by the allure of the drink, but by the overwhelming weight of distress? This might come as a surprise, but distress, both emotional and physical, plays a pivotal role in the journey of recovery.

In this chapter, we'll delve deep into the intricate relationship between distress and alcoholism. We'll explore the different types of distress, understand their signs, and evaluate their impact on the recovery process. Furthermore, we'll introduce you to the DBT techniques specifically designed to manage and alleviate these distresses. By the end of this chapter, you'll be equipped with practical tools and insights to handle distress effectively, enhancing your resilience against potential relapses.

Distress, in its many forms, is a silent saboteur in the journey of re-covery. Emotional distress, often stemming from past traumas, unre-solved conflicts, or daily life pressures, can push an individual towards alcohol as a temporary escape. On the other hand, physical distress, which can arise from withdrawal symptoms or other health issues, can also act as a potent trigger. Recognizing the signs of distress is the first step. It's like identifying the enemy before devising a strategy. The journey of recovery is not just about staying away from alcohol; it's also about understanding and managing the myriad factors, like distress, that influence the urge to drink.

DBT, with its roots in cognitive behavioral therapy, offers a robust set of tools to handle distress. The acceptance and change strategies em-power individuals to accept their current state while working towards a positive change. Crisis survival strategies are like the emergency tools one needs when caught in a storm, helping to navigate through intense bouts of distress without resorting to alcohol. Self-soothing techniques, on the other hand, are preventive measures, ensuring that the distress doesn't escalate in the first place.

To truly grasp the efficacy of DBT in managing distress, let's consider some real-life scenarios. Imagine Sarah, a 28-year-old who recently lost her job. The emotional turmoil, combined with the pressures of unpaid bills, pushes her towards the brink of relapse. But, equipped with the DBT techniques, she recognizes her emotional distress signs and employs self-soothing techniques, such as deep breathing and mindfulness, to navigate through the crisis. Similarly, role plays and reflective anecdotes from various individuals will further illuminate the practical application of DBT in diverse distressing situations.

Emotional distress is a complex beast, often lurking in the shadows, waiting for a vulnerable moment to strike. It's not just about feeling sad or upset; it's a profound sense of unease, a turmoil that can shake one's very foundation. For many recovering from alcoholism, these emotional upheavals can be the very triggers that push them back into the abyss of addiction.

Historically, societies have often downplayed the significance of emotional well-being, focusing more on physical health. But as we've evolved in our understanding, we've come to realize that emotional health is just as crucial, if not more so. In the context of alcoholism, emotional distress can arise from various sources - unresolved past traumas, the strain of daily life, or even the anxiety of the recovery process itself.

Marsha Linehan, the pioneer behind DBT, emphasized the importance of recognizing and addressing emotional distress. She believed that by understanding our emotional triggers, we could develop strategies to cope with them without resorting to self-destructive behaviors like excessive drinking. Through DBT, she introduced techniques that help individuals sit with their distress, understand it, and then take proactive steps to alleviate it.

Resilience is often seen as an innate trait, something you're either born with or without. But in reality, resilience is like a muscle; it can be developed and strengthened over time. Through DBT, individuals can build their emotional resilience, ensuring that they can face life's challenges head-on without resorting to alcohol.

This involves a combination of acceptance strategies, where one learns to accept their current emotional state, and change strategies, where one works towards a positive emotional shift. It's about understanding that while we can't always control our emotions, we can control our reactions to them.

While understanding the theory behind DBT is essential, its real power lies in its practical application. This means incorporating DBT techniques into daily life, making them a part of one's routine. Whether it's starting the day with a mindfulness exercise, journaling about one's emotions, or employing crisis survival strategies when faced with a particularly challenging situation, the consistent application of DBT can make a significant difference in one's recovery journey.

At its core, alcoholism is as much an emotional issue as it is a physical one. The bottle becomes a refuge, a place to hide from pain, from trauma, from the everyday stresses of life. But in doing so, it also becomes a barrier, a wall that separates the individual from their loved ones. Conversations become confrontations, intimacy turns into isolation.

Imagine a scenario where a husband comes home late, reeking of alcohol. His wife, worried, asks him where he's been. Instead of responding, he lashes out, angry, defensive. This isn't the man she married, but the alcohol speaking. Over time, these incidents accumulate, eroding the foundation of their relationship.

Recovery isn't a one-time event; it's a continuous process. And the same goes for mending relationships. It's not about grand gestures but consistent, small acts that show one's commitment to change. This might mean regularly attending therapy sessions, joining a support group, or simply setting aside time each day for self-reflection.

In the world of DBT, there's a concept called 'wise mind'. It's the intersection of emotional mind and reasonable mind, a balance between feeling and thinking. In the journey of recovery, tapping into one's wise mind can be invaluable. It's about recognizing and respecting one's emotions while also making rational, informed decisions.

In the midst of the storm that is addiction, it's easy to lose oneself. The person staring back in the mirror seems like a stranger, a shadow of who they once were. But herein lies a potent tool for recovery: self-reflection.

Every action, every choice, has a reason behind it. For many battling addiction, drinking isn't just about the physical craving but the emotional void it fills, even if momentarily. By delving deep into oneself, by asking the hard questions, one can begin to understand the 'why' behind their actions. Why does a stressful day at work lead to a night of binge drinking? Why does an argument with a loved one result in turning to the bottle?

Dialectical Behavior Therapy, with its emphasis on mindfulness, offers a structured path to this self-exploration. It's not about judging oneself but observing. Observing without criticism, without bias. It's about understanding one's triggers, one's patterns.

Imagine a scenario where every time someone feels rejected, they turn to alcohol. Through DBT, they can learn to recognize this pattern, to understand the deep-seated fear of rejection that drives this behavior. And in this recognition lies the first step to change.

Certainly! Let's replace the journaling takeaway with a focus on the role of distress in alcoholism and how DBT techniques can be pivotal in managing it.

The journey of recovery, as depicted in the chapter, is not just about abstaining from alcohol but understanding oneself deeply. This introspection, this deep dive into one's psyche, is the cornerstone of lasting recovery. It's about recognizing patterns, understanding triggers, and then using this knowledge to make informed choices.:

The chapter emphasized the importance of understanding the 'why' behind our actions. This isn't a superficial exploration but a profound understanding of the deep-seated emotions and triggers that lead to certain behaviors. For someone battling addiction, this understanding can be the difference between relapse and recovery.

Dialectical Behavior Therapy isn't just another therapeutic approach. It's a structured path to self-awareness. Its emphasis on mindfulness, on non-judgmental observation, offers individuals a way to understand their patterns without the cloud of self-criticism. This non-judgmental stance is crucial because it allows for genuine introspection without the barriers of guilt or shame.

One of the most profound revelations from the chapter was understanding the role of distress in alcoholism. Distress, both emotional and physical, can act as a silent aggravator, pushing individuals towards relapse. Recognizing and managing this distress becomes pivotal, and DBT offers the tools to do just that.

Recovery isn't a sprint; it's a marathon. And just like any long journey, consistency is key. The chapter emphasized the importance of regular self-reflection, of consistently using tools like DBT techniques to stay on the path of recovery.

While the chapter delved deep into self-reflection and its role in recovery, it also highlighted the bigger picture. Recovery isn't just about the individual but also about their relationships, their place in the world. And as we move forward, understanding this bigger picture becomes crucial.

Now that we have covered the realm of distress tolerance, we've come to recognize its paramount importance in the recovery journey. Mastering distress tolerance isn't just about navigating the stormy seas of immediate crises; it's about equipping oneself with the tools to sail smoothly even when the waters are calm, but the undercurrents are unpredictable. As we've seen, it's these unseen undercurrents, the silent triggers, and the unaddressed distress, that can often steer one off course. But what happens once we've learned to recognize and manage this distress? How does this mastery impact our interactions with the world around us, especially our relationships that might have been strained due to past behaviors? In the next chapter, we'll take a look at what the pathway to recovery looks like and why the structure of recovery is as crucial as it is.

# Chapter Seven

---

# Structuring Success: The Power of Planning in Recovery

"In the unpredictable journey of recovery, the most consistent ally is often the structure we build for ourselves."

In this chapter, we'll delve into the transformative power of structure in the recovery process. From its role in preventing relapse to the mental health benefits it offers, structure acts as the backbone of a successful recovery journey. We'll also explore how DBT aids in building a personalized recovery plan and the importance of staying accountable through various means.

When we talk about recovery, especially from something as gripping as alcoholism, the journey is often visualized as a path filled with obstacles, challenges, and moments of self-doubt. In this tumultuous journey, structure stands as a beacon, a guiding light that offers direction and purpose.

Relapse, the dreaded word in the world of recovery, often lurks in the shadows of unstructured time. When the mind is idle, it tends to wander, and for someone battling addiction, it often wanders to the very thing they're trying to avoid. Structure, in this context, acts as a protective shield. By filling one's day with purposeful activities, there's less room for the mind to stray. It's akin to having a map in a dense forest. While the path might still be challenging, the chances of getting lost are significantly reduced. This structure doesn't just mean filling up one's day with random activities; it's about meaningful engagement that aligns with one's recovery goals.

Beyond relapse prevention, structure offers a plethora of benefits for mental health. Humans, by nature, are creatures of habit. We thrive on routine and predictability. When our days have a rhythm, a certain flow, it instills a sense of normalcy, which can be incredibly grounding, especially during the early stages of recovery. Each task completed, each goal achieved, adds to a sense of accomplishment. Over time, these small victories accumulate, bolstering self-esteem and fostering a positive self-image.

However, it's essential to understand that structure isn't a one-size-fits-all solution. What might work for one individual could be counterproductive for another. This is where personalization comes into play. Crafting a structure that aligns with one's unique needs, challenges, and goals is paramount. It's about striking a balance between rigidity and flexibility, ensuring that while there's a routine in place, there's also room for spontaneity and adaptability.

Dialectical Behavior Therapy (DBT) is more than just a therapeutic approach; it's a philosophy, a way of life that emphasizes balance, acceptance, and change. Integrating DBT into one's recovery plan can be transformative.

Before diving into the techniques and strategies that DBT offers, it's crucial to take a step back and assess where one stands. This self-assessment is a deep, introspective process. It's about understanding one's triggers, recognizing strengths, and acknowledging areas that need attention. This isn't a one-off process. As one progresses in their recovery journey, their needs, challenges, and strengths evolve. Regular reassessments ensure that the recovery plan remains dynamic, adapting to these changes.

Our surroundings play a significant role in our mental well-being. For someone in recovery, creating a safe, alcohol-free environment is paramount. This might mean decluttering one's living space, removing any alcohol or related paraphernalia, and creating dedicated spaces for relaxation, reflection, and self-care.

Routine brings predictability, and predictability can be comforting. Establishing a daily routine, which includes time for self-care, work, hobbies, and social connections, can provide a sense of purpose and direction. This routine acts as a roadmap, guiding individuals through their day and minimizing the chances of encountering unexpected triggers.

Physical activity, whether it's a brisk walk, yoga, or a gym session, offers a plethora of benefits. It releases endorphins, the body's natural feel-good chemicals, reduces stress, and improves sleep quality. Incorporating regular physical activity into one's routine can act as a natural mood booster, supporting mental well-being.

With a clear understanding of one's current state, the next step is goal setting. But these aren't just any goals; they're SMART - Specific, Measurable, Achievable, Relevant, and Time-bound. Whether it's staying sober for a month, mending a strained relationship, or picking up a new hobby, each goal should be clear and actionable. These goals act as milestones, markers that offer direction and purpose.

However, even the best-laid plans can go awry. This is where reflection comes into play. Regularly reviewing one's recovery plan, celebrating the successes, learning from the missteps, and tweaking the plan accordingly is essential. It ensures that the plan remains relevant, effective, and aligned with one's evolving needs.

Accountability, in the world of recovery, is a powerful tool. It's about taking ownership of one's journey, being responsible for one's actions, and being answerable to oneself and others.

In the realm of accountability, support groups play a pivotal role. These groups, whether formal or informal, offer a sense of community, a space where individuals can share their stories, challenges, and victories. But beyond that, they offer a platform for mutual accountability. Knowing that there are others who are invested in your recovery, who are cheering for you, can be incredibly motivating. It's a reminder that one isn't alone in this journey.

In today's digital age, there are myriad tools available, from mobile apps to journals, that can help individuals track their progress. Documenting one's journey, the highs, the lows, the challenges, and the victories, offers a tangible record of how far one has come. On challenging days, revisiting these records can offer solace and motivation.

Recovery is a journey filled with milestones, both big and small. Celebrating these milestones, whether it's a month of sobriety or successfully navigating a particularly challenging trigger, is essential. These celebrations aren't just about marking an achievement; they're about recognizing the hard work, resilience, and determination that went into reaching that milestone.

Addiction can strain relationships, leading to feelings of isolation and loneliness. DBT emphasizes the importance of interpersonal effectiveness, which is about building and nurturing healthy relationships. It's about effective communication, setting boundaries, and seeking and offering support.

Recovery is a journey, not a destination. It's about continuous growth, learning, and adaptation. As one chapter closes, another begins, filled with new challenges, opportunities, and victories.

The world of addiction and recovery is ever-evolving, with new research, therapies, and insights emerging regularly. Embracing a mindset of continuous learning ensures that one remains updated, equipped with the latest tools and strategies to support their recovery journey.

No one is an island, and this is particularly true in recovery. Building a support system, whether it's family, friends, therapists, or support groups, can be a game-changer. It's about having a safety net, a group of individuals who understand, support, and cheer for you.

The future is uncertain, filled with unknowns. For someone in recovery, this uncertainty can be daunting. But it's essential to embrace the unknown, to see it not as a challenge but as an opportunity. It's about taking each day as it comes, celebrating the victories, learning from the setbacks, and always, always moving forward.

One of the core principles of DBT is radical acceptance, which is about accepting life as it is, without judgment. For someone in recovery, this means accepting their past, their challenges, and their current reality. It's about letting go of guilt, shame, and self-blame and focusing on the present and the future.

The journey of recovery is akin to navigating a ship through turbulent waters. Without a compass or a map, the ship is at the mercy of the waves, vulnerable to being thrown off course. Structure, in the context of recovery, serves as that compass, that map. It provides direction, stability, and a sense of purpose. It's not just about setting a daily routine; it's about creating an environment and a lifestyle that nurtures sobriety and well-being.

Our surroundings have a profound impact on our mental and emotional state. A cluttered, chaotic environment can exacerbate feelings of anxiety and overwhelm. On the other hand, a serene, organized space can promote calmness and clarity. For someone on the path of recovery, curating a conducive environment is not a luxury; it's a necessity. It's about creating a sanctuary, a safe haven where one can heal, reflect, and grow.

The mind-body connection is undeniable. Physical activity, be it a gentle yoga session or an invigorating run, offers manifold benefits. It acts as a natural stress-reliever, releasing a surge of endorphins, the body's feel-good chemicals. Moreover, it serves as a constructive outlet, a way to channel and process emotions. For someone grappling with addiction, physical activity can be a lifeline, a way to reconnect with their body and rediscover its strength and resilience.

Dialectical Behavior Therapy (DBT) is more than just a therapeutic approach; it's a philosophy, a way of life. It equips individuals with tools and strategies to navigate the complexities of life. Radical acceptance, for instance, teaches the art of embracing life, with all its imperfections. It's about letting go of resistance, of the "should haves" and "could haves," and finding peace in the present. Similarly, the emphasis on interpersonal effectiveness underscores the importance of healthy, nurturing relationships in the recovery journey.

Recovery is not a destination; it's a journey, one that demands continuous growth, learning, and adaptation. The world of addiction and recovery is dynamic, with new research and insights emerging regularly. Adopting a mindset of lifelong learning ensures that one remains equipped to face the challenges that lie ahead. It's about being proactive, staying updated, and always striving for better.

Humans are inherently social beings, craving connection and belonging. In the context of recovery, the role of community and support cannot be overstated. Whether it's family, friends, therapists, or support groups, having a robust support system can make all the difference. It's about having a tribe, a group of individuals who understand, empathize, and uplift.

The future, with all its uncertainties, can be daunting. Yet, it's essential to approach it with hope, optimism, and an open heart. It's about seeing challenges as opportunities, setbacks as lessons. With the right tools, strategies, and mindset, the future is not something to be feared, but to be embraced.

Having journeyed through the structured pathways of recovery and the transformative power of DBT, we stand at the precipice of a topic that many in recovery often find daunting: setbacks and relapses. It's a natural progression from understanding the foundational structures to addressing the inevitable challenges that arise on this journey. The path to sobriety isn't always a straight one; it's filled with twists, turns, and sometimes, regressions. But these moments, as challenging as they may be, offer invaluable lessons and insights.

In our upcoming chapter, "Overcoming Setbacks and Relapses," we will delve deep into the heart of these challenges. We'll explore the psychological and emotional underpinnings of relapses, understand their triggers, and most importantly, equip ourselves with strategies to rise again with renewed vigor. It's about understanding that setbacks are not failures but are instead stepping stones, each one carving a deeper, more resilient path towards lasting recovery. As we transition, remember that every chapter in our recovery journey, including the challenging ones, contributes to our overarching narrative of strength, resilience, and hope.

# Chapter Eight

---

# Overcoming Setbacks and Relapses

The room was dimly lit, with the faint aroma of burnt candles. Sarah sat on her couch, staring blankly at the empty bottle on the table. It had been six months since her last drink. But tonight, the weight of the world had been too much. Tears streamed down her face as she thought of the progress she had lost. But little did she know, this setback was about to become the cornerstone of her recovery, all thanks to the principles of DBT.

Relapses are often viewed as the end of the road in the recovery journey. But in reality, they're just a detour, a momentary lapse that can be overcome with the right tools and mindset. In this chapter, we'll delve deep into understanding relapses, the role of DBT in navigating them, and how to move forward with renewed determination.

Relapses are not just about returning to a previous behavior; they're a complex interplay of emotions, triggers, and circumstances. Often, they're precipitated by a combination of internal and external factors, from personal stressors to environmental cues. For someone recovering from alcoholism, even the clink of glasses or the smell of alcohol can act as a trigger. It's essential to recognize these triggers and understand the underlying emotions they evoke.

The emotional aftermath of a relapse can be overwhelming. Feelings of guilt, shame, and disappointment often cloud the individual's judgment, making them question their entire recovery journey. However, it's crucial to remember that recovery is not a linear path. It's filled with ups and downs, and each setback offers a unique learning opportunity.

The journey back to recovery post-relapse begins with acceptance. Accepting that relapses can happen, understanding the reasons behind it, and being compassionate towards oneself are the first steps. It's not about how many times one falls, but how many times they get back up, armed with more knowledge and determination than before.

DBT, with its emphasis on emotional regulation and mindfulness, offers a beacon of hope post-relapse. The techniques taught in DBT, such as distress tolerance and radical acceptance, can be instrumental in navigating the emotional storm that follows a relapse. By grounding oneself in the present moment and accepting the situation without judgment, one can start the healing process.

Post-relapse, emotions can be in turmoil. DBT offers tools to recognize these emotions without getting overwhelmed by them. Techniques like deep breathing, mindfulness meditation, and guided imagery can help regain emotional balance, providing a clear headspace to plan the next steps in recovery.

A relapse can often lead to broken trust, both in oneself and in relationships with loved ones. Using DBT's interpersonal effectiveness strategies, one can work on rebuilding this trust. It's about open communication, understanding the other person's perspective, and making amends.

Every setback offers a chance to re-evaluate one's goals. Post-relapse, it's essential to reflect on what went wrong and set new, realistic goals. Whether it's attending more therapy sessions, joining a support group, or practicing DBT techniques daily, these goals act as a roadmap for the recovery journey ahead.

Recovery is not a journey one has to undertake alone. Post-relapse, seeking additional support, be it from therapists, support groups, or loved ones, can make a world of difference. Sharing one's feelings, fears, and hopes can provide a fresh perspective and renewed motivation.

Consistency is key in recovery. Regularly practicing DBT techniques, journaling about one's experiences, and reflecting on the progress can reinforce the learnings and make them second nature.

Opening up about a relapse can be one of the most challenging steps in the recovery process. The fear of judgment, the weight of disappointment, and the vulnerability it brings can be daunting. Yet, there's immense power in vulnerability. By sharing one's story, not only does one unburden themselves, but they also pave the way for others to understand and offer support.

Imagine a tree, standing tall and proud. A storm comes, and a branch breaks. The tree doesn't hide the broken branch; it stands there, exposed, allowing the world to see its imperfection. With time, around the broken branch, new sprouts emerge, making the tree even more robust and more resilient. Similarly, by acknowledging and sharing our relapses, we allow ourselves to grow stronger, with deeper roots in our recovery journey.

No person is an island. Especially in recovery, the community plays a pivotal role. Whether it's a support group, a therapist, or loved ones, having a community to lean on can make the journey less daunting. They act as a mirror, reflecting our progress, our setbacks, and offering a fresh perspective when we're too close to the problem.

Think of it as trekking up a mountain. Alone, the journey can be overwhelming. But with a group, there's shared responsibility. When one person falters, another offers a hand. When one loses their way, another points to the path. The journey becomes a shared experience, filled with collective memories, challenges, and triumphs.

Often, post-relapse, the harshest critic is oneself. The internal dialogue can be debilitating, filled with self-blame and regret. Here's where the principles of DBT come into play, emphasizing the importance of self-compassion. It's about treating oneself with the same kindness and understanding as one would treat a dear friend.

Imagine a child learning to ride a bike. They wobble, they fall, they get a few scrapes. Would we scold them for falling? Or would we encourage them to get back on, praising their effort and determination? The same approach is needed for oneself post-relapse. Recognizing the effort, understanding the challenges, and encouraging oneself to keep moving forward.

Relapse isn't a singular event but often a cycle, a dance between recovery and setback. Understanding this cycle is crucial because it helps in recognizing patterns, triggers, and vulnerabilities. It's not about labeling oneself as a failure but about understanding the nuances of one's journey.

Imagine the ebb and flow of the ocean. The waves come crashing to the shore, only to retreat and come back again. This rhythm is natural, just as the rhythm of relapse and recovery can be for many. The key is not to fight against the current but to learn how to navigate it, to ride the waves with skill and grace.

The emotional aftermath of a relapse can be more challenging than the physical one. Feelings of guilt, shame, and self-doubt can cloud one's judgment, making it harder to return to the path of recovery. It's essential to address these emotions, not bury them, for they hold the key to understanding oneself better.

Consider a wound. If left untreated, it can fester and become infected. But with the right care, it heals, leaving behind a scar—a testament to resilience and healing. Similarly, addressing the emotional wounds post-relapse can lead to profound healing and understanding.

Recovery isn't a static state but a dynamic process. It evolves, changes, and adapts, just as we do. Recognizing this dynamism can be empowering. It means that every day offers a new opportunity, a fresh start, a chance to redefine one's journey.

Think of a river, constantly flowing, changing course, adapting to the landscape. There are calm stretches, turbulent rapids, and meandering turns. Yet, the river never stops; it keeps flowing. Similarly, the journey of recovery, with its calm moments and challenges, is continuous, ever-evolving.

One of the most potent tools in the recovery toolkit is forgiveness—not just forgiving others but oneself. Relapse can often lead to feelings of self-blame and resentment. But holding onto these emotions can be a roadblock in the recovery journey. Forgiveness, on the other hand, can be liberating.

Imagine holding onto a heavy backpack while trying to climb a mountain. The weight slows you down, making the climb more challenging. Letting go of this backpack, filled with guilt and resentment, can make the journey lighter and more manageable. Forgiveness is that act of letting go, allowing oneself to move forward with a lighter heart.

As we transition from understanding the intricacies of relapse and recovery, the next chapter, "Overcoming Setbacks and Relapses," will provide a deeper exploration into practical strategies and insights. It will guide readers on how to turn challenges into stepping stones, ensuring that every setback becomes a setup for a comeback.

Recovery is not just about the end goal of sobriety; it's about the journey. Every step, every challenge, every triumph is a part of the process. By embracing the journey, one learns to find joy in the small victories, understanding in the setbacks, and growth in the challenges.

Consider a mosaic - a piece of art made up of broken pieces. Each piece, with its unique shape, size, and color, comes together to create something beautiful. Similarly, our recovery journey, with its ups and downs, comes together to create a life filled with purpose, understanding, and resilience.

The journey of recovery is akin to a dance, a rhythmic ebb and flow between progress and setbacks. Just as a dancer learns to move with grace, adapting to the rhythm of the music, individuals on the path of recovery learn to navigate the challenges and triumphs of their journey. The dance is not about perfection but about resilience, understanding, and growth.

Relapse is not an isolated incident but part of a broader cycle. Recognizing this cycle is pivotal. It's about discerning patterns, triggers, and vulnerabilities. The ocean's waves, with their relentless ebb and flow, serve as a metaphor for this cycle. The key lies not in resisting the waves but in learning to ride them, understanding their rhythm, and using it to one's advantage.

The emotional toll of a relapse can often overshadow its physical repercussions. Feelings of guilt, shame, and self-doubt can be overwhelming. However, these emotions, when addressed and processed, can lead to profound self-awareness and understanding. Like a wound that heals to leave a scar, these emotional scars can be reminders of resilience, growth, and the ability to overcome.

Recovery is not a destination but a journey—a dynamic, ever-evolving process. This journey is filled with opportunities, fresh starts, and moments of introspection. Like a river that never stops flowing, changing its course as it encounters obstacles, the journey of recovery is about adaptability, persistence, and the will to keep moving forward.

In the recovery journey, forgiveness emerges as a potent tool. It's not just about forgiving others but, more importantly, forgiving oneself.

Holding onto guilt and resentment can be burdensome, hindering progress. In contrast, forgiveness lightens the soul, making the path to recovery smoother and more manageable. It's the act of releasing the heavy baggage of the past to move forward with hope and determination.

Having journeyed through the tumultuous waters of relapse and recovery, we stand at a pivotal juncture. The past chapters have illuminated the challenges and emotional roller-coasters that accompany the path to sobriety. But as the horizon of recovery stretches out before us, a new question emerges: How do we ensure that this newfound sobriety stands the test of time? How do we fortify ourselves against the siren calls of old habits and temptations?

The dance of recovery, as we've seen, is intricate, filled with highs and lows. But as any seasoned dancer knows, the key to a flawless performance isn't just in mastering individual steps but in sustaining the rhythm over the long haul. The upcoming chapter, "Maintaining Sobriety: Long-Term Strategies," seeks to be that guiding rhythm. It aims to equip readers with the tools, strategies, and mindsets necessary to not just achieve sobriety, but to maintain it as a lifelong commitment. We'll delve into the art of building resilience, fortifying our mental and emotional defenses, and cultivating an environment conducive to sustained recovery. The journey ahead promises to be enlightening, offering a roadmap to a life of continued sobriety and fulfillment.

# Chapter Nine

---

# Maintaining Sobriety: Long-Term Strategies

"Recovery is not a destination, but a journey that evolves with each sunrise."

The path to sobriety is not a sprint but a marathon, a lifelong journey that requires dedication, resilience, and continuous growth. In this chapter, we'll delve deep into understanding the evolving nature of recovery, the importance of incorporating DBT into daily life, and the significance of building a robust support system. Through stories, techniques, and insights, we'll explore the tools needed to maintain long-term sobriety and thrive.

Recovery is not a static state but a dynamic process. Just as life changes, so does one's journey in sobriety. It's essential to recognize that recovery evolves, adapting to life's challenges and joys. Over time, the reasons for staying sober might shift, and the strategies that once worked might need revisiting. Embracing this fluidity can be the key to enduring success.

While the initial stages of recovery come with their hurdles, long-term sobriety presents its unique set of challenges. From complacency to external pressures, understanding these challenges can equip individuals to navigate them effectively. It's crucial to remember that every stage of recovery has its lessons and growth opportunities.

Narratives have the power to inspire and motivate. By exploring stories of those who've maintained sobriety over the years, readers can glean insights, hope, and strategies that resonate with their journey. These tales serve as a testament to the strength of the human spirit and the transformative power of sustained recovery.

Mindfulness, like we covered earlier, is the art of being present and is a cornerstone in maintaining sobriety. By incorporating daily practices like mindful breathing, meditation, or even mindful eating, individuals can cultivate a heightened sense of awareness, making it easier to navigate triggers and stressors.

Emotions, if unchecked, can become overwhelming. By continuously practicing emotional regulation techniques learned through DBT, one can ensure that they respond to life's ups and downs in a balanced and healthy manner. This might involve revisiting DBT exercises or even seeking advanced techniques as one progresses in their journey.

The path to sobriety is one of continuous growth. By setting aside time for regular self-reflection, individuals can assess their progress, recognize areas of improvement, and celebrate milestones. These check-ins can be daily, weekly, or even monthly, but they serve as a grounding ritual in the recovery journey.

While personal strength is vital, the role of external support cannot be understated. Therapy and support groups offer a safe space to share, learn, and grow. They provide a sense of community, a reminder that one is not alone in their journey.

Relationships play a pivotal role in recovery. From friends and family to mentors and peers in recovery, these interpersonal connections offer emotional support, guidance, and a sense of belonging. Nurturing these relationships can be the bedrock of sustained sobriety.

Recovery is a journey of continuous learning. By seeking ongoing education, be it through books, workshops, or seminars, individuals can equip themselves with the latest strategies and insights in the realm of recovery. This commitment to growth ensures that one remains proactive in their sobriety journey.

That said, it's very important to note that recovery is also an ongoing process of self-discovery and growth. Embracing continuous learning means staying updated with new research, techniques, and strategies that can aid in sobriety. Attending workshops, reading books, or even participating in online forums can provide fresh insights and perspectives.

As one progresses in their recovery journey, understanding and setting boundaries becomes crucial. This might involve distancing oneself from certain individuals, avoiding specific environments, or even setting time boundaries to ensure self-care. Clear boundaries protect one's mental and emotional well-being, ensuring that the recovery journey remains uninterrupted.

Financial stress can be a significant trigger for many. Ensuring financial stability involves creating a budget, managing debts, and seeking financial counseling if needed. Being financially secure can reduce anxiety and provide a sense of control, both of which are beneficial for long-term sobriety.

For many, the journey of recovery is also a spiritual one. Exploring spirituality doesn't necessarily mean adhering to a particular religion. It could be about understanding one's place in the universe, meditating, or even connecting with nature. This spiritual connection can offer solace, purpose, and a deeper understanding of oneself.

What we consume can significantly impact our mental and emotional state. A balanced diet, rich in nutrients, can boost mood, energy levels, and overall well-being. Understanding the role of nutrition, and perhaps even consulting with a nutritionist, can be an essential step in the recovery journey.

Traveling can be therapeutic. It offers a change of environment, exposes one to new cultures, and provides a break from routine. However, it's essential to plan trips carefully to avoid potential triggers. Choosing sober travel groups, planning activities in advance, and ensuring one has access to support, even while traveling, can make journeys enjoyable and relapse-free.

Recovery is a journey, not a destination. This chapter has illuminated the multifaceted nature of maintaining sobriety, emphasizing that it's not just about abstaining from alcohol but about building a life where alcohol no longer holds a place. Here are the pivotal insights we've gleaned:

1. The Evolving Nature of Recovery: Sobriety isn't a static state but a dynamic process. As life changes, so do the challenges and joys of recovery. Embracing this fluidity allows individuals to adapt, grow, and find renewed purpose at every stage of their journey.

2. Continuous Learning: Recovery is also about evolving as a person. By staying updated with new research, techniques, and strategies, individuals can equip themselves with the latest tools to aid their sobriety journey, ensuring they remain resilient in the face of new challenges.

3. The Power of Boundaries: Recovery often means re-evaluating relationships and environments. Setting clear boundaries—whether with people, places, or personal habits—ensures that one's mental and emotional well-being remains protected.

4. Financial Stability: Financial stress can be a silent trigger. Achieving financial stability, be it through budgeting, managing debts, or seeking counseling, can significantly reduce anxiety, offering a clearer path to sustained sobriety.

5. Nutrition's Role: The mind-body connection is undeniable. A balanced diet can bolster mental health, providing the energy and mood stability crucial for those in recovery. It's not just about what we abstain from but also what we consume that shapes our recovery journey.

6. Travel as Therapy: While travel offers a refreshing break, it's essential to approach it with mindfulness. Planning trips with sobriety

in mind—like choosing sober travel groups or planning activities in advance—ensures that the journey rejuvenates rather than triggers.

7. Spiritual Exploration: For many, recovery intertwines with spirituality. This exploration, whether through organized religion, meditation, or nature, can offer a deeper understanding of oneself, providing solace and purpose.

8. DBT's Daily Role: Dialectical Behavior Therapy isn't just a treatment—it's a lifestyle. Incorporating its principles daily, from mindfulness practices to regular reflections, ensures that the foundation of recovery remains robust.

9. Support Systems: No one recovers alone. Building and maintaining a support system, be it through therapy, support groups, or interpersonal relationships, is paramount. These networks offer guidance, accountability, and the reminder that one is never alone in their journey.

10. Looking Ahead: Recovery is about the past, present, and future. While it's essential to address past traumas and stay grounded in the present, looking ahead is equally crucial. Setting new goals, seeking additional support, and reinforcing DBT practices ensures that the path to sobriety remains clear and focused.

As we reflect upon the intricate tapestry of recovery, it's evident that sobriety is more than just the absence of alcohol—it's a transformative journey that reshapes every facet of one's life. The strategies and insights we've delved into in this chapter lay the groundwork for a life of sustained sobriety. However, the principles of Dialectical Behavior Therapy (DBT) are not just tools for recovery; they are guiding lights for a fulfilling, balanced life.

The next chapter, "Beyond Alcohol Recovery: Living a DBT-Informed Life," will broaden our horizons further. We'll explore how the core principles of DBT can be seamlessly integrated into daily life, not just as a reactive measure against potential relapses but as a proactive approach to cultivate emotional well-being, resilience, and genuine happiness. We'll delve into the profound ways DBT can influence our relationships, our career choices, our daily routines, and even the manner in which we perceive the world around us.

Imagine a life where challenges are met with grace, where emotional turbulence is navigated with skill, and where every moment is lived with mindfulness and purpose. That's the promise of a DBT-informed life—a life beyond mere recovery, a life of profound fulfillment and balance. Join us as we embark on this transformative journey, taking the principles of DBT from the realm of recovery to the vast expanse of everyday living.

# Chapter Ten

---

# Beyond Alcohol Recovery: Living a DBT-Informed Life

H ave you ever pondered how the skills learned in one area of life can ripple out, influencing various facets of your existence? What if the tools you acquired to combat addiction could also be your guiding light in navigating the intricate maze of daily life?

In this chapter, we'll explore the expansive horizon of Dialectical Behavior Therapy (DBT) beyond the confines of addiction recovery. We'll delve into its broader applications, from enhancing emotional intelligence in relationships to managing everyday distress. Through inspiring life stories, we'll witness the transformative power of DBT in personal growth and its potential to create a ripple effect, touching not just the individual but the community at large.

The universality of DBT is not limited to addiction. Its principles, rooted in the balance of acceptance and change, are applicable in various scenarios. Whether it's the stress of a looming deadline, the anxiety of a first date, or the frustration of a traffic jam, DBT offers tools to navigate these with grace and composure.

Enhancing one's emotional intelligence is a journey, not a destination. With DBT, this journey is enriched. It's about understanding your emotions, recognizing triggers, and responding rather than reacting. It's about listening, truly listening, to a loved one's concerns without judgment. It's about expressing oneself clearly, assertively, and compassionately.

Daily life is filled with challenges, both big and small. From the morning rush to the evening wind-down, moments of distress are inevitable. But with DBT, these moments become opportunities. Opportunities to practice mindfulness, to apply distress tolerance techniques, or to engage in effective communication.

Relationships, whether familial, romantic, or platonic, are the bedrock of our social existence. They bring joy, support, and love. But they can also bring conflict, misunderstanding, and pain. DBT, with its emphasis on emotional regulation and interpersonal effectiveness, offers a roadmap to healthier, more fulfilling relationships.

Life stories are testament to the transformative power of DBT. Take, for instance, the story of Maya. A recovering alcoholic, Maya found solace in DBT not just for her addiction, but for her daily life. From managing her anxiety at work to improving her relationship with her teenage daughter, DBT became her compass.

Growth is an ongoing process. It doesn't stop once a particular milestone is achieved. With DBT, this journey is continuous. It's about setting new goals, reflecting on one's progress, and adapting as needed. It's about lifelong learning and self-improvement.

Challenges are a part of this journey. But with DBT, they become manageable. Whether it's a relapse, a personal loss, or a global pandemic, DBT offers strategies to navigate these with resilience and strength.

Sharing is caring. And when it comes to DBT, sharing its principles can be transformative. Whether it's introducing a friend to mindfulness meditation, guiding a loved one through a distress tolerance exercise, or simply being a listening ear, spreading the knowledge of DBT can have a ripple effect.

Building a community of support is essential. This could be in the form of therapy groups, support groups, or simply a close-knit group of friends and family. Such a community offers a safe space to practice DBT skills, to share experiences, and to seek guidance.

Advocacy and awareness are crucial. By spreading the word about DBT, by sharing its success stories, and by advocating for its inclusion in recovery programs, we can bring about a change. A change not just in the lives of individuals, but in the fabric of society.

Mindfulness, a word you're probably oh so sick of hearing by now. Well it's your lucky day because I'll only be going on one more rant about it and that happens to be right now. If there's anything you should take from me preaching the word "mindfulness" all throughout this book it's the fact that mindfulness is a cornerstone of DBT. It isn't just for the therapy room. It's a practice that can be woven into the fabric of our daily lives, transforming mundane tasks into moments of presence and awareness. Please take these following things into consideration when the word mindfulness pops into your brain at any given time.

In a world of fast food and faster lives, taking the time to truly savor our meals can be a revolutionary act. Mindful eating is about appreciating the colors, textures, and flavors of our food. It's about listening to our body's hunger and fullness cues, and recognizing the emotions that often drive our eating habits.

Whether it's a stroll in the park or the daily walk to the subway station, walking can be an act of mindfulness. It's about feeling the ground beneath our feet, noticing the rhythm of our breath, and truly being present in the moment.

In an age of digital distractions, truly listening to someone has become a rare gift. Mindful listening is about being fully present with the speaker, without judgment or distraction. It's about understanding, not just hearing.

While DBT equips us with tools and strategies to navigate the challenges of life, it also emphasizes the importance of treating ourselves with kindness and compassion.

At its core, self-compassion is about treating ourselves with the same kindness, concern, and understanding that we'd offer to a good friend. It's about recognizing our shared humanity, and understanding that everyone, including us, is doing the best they can with the resources they have.

While self-esteem is about evaluating ourselves positively, self-compassion is about relating to ourselves kindly. It's not about puffing ourselves up, but about being gentle with ourselves, especially in moments of failure or inadequacy.

From loving-kindness meditations to self-compassion journaling, there are numerous practices that can help us cultivate a kinder, gentler relationship with ourselves. These practices not only enhance our emotional well-being but also strengthen our resilience in the face of challenges.

The journey of recovery, as we've explored in Chapter 10, is not just about overcoming addiction but about embracing a fuller, more present way of living. Here are the key takeaways that illuminate the path forward:

1. The Power of Mindfulness in Daily Activities: Mindfulness is not a fleeting concept confined to meditation sessions. It's a way of life. When we eat, we can savor every bite, appreciating the nourishment and flavors. When we walk, whether it's amidst nature or in a bustling city, we can feel the ground beneath, the air around, and the rhythm of our heartbeats. And when we listen, we can truly hear, understanding the unsaid and feeling the emotions beneath the words. This daily mindfulness transforms ordinary moments into extraordinary experiences.

2. DBT Beyond Therapy: Dialectical Behavior Therapy (DBT) is not just a therapeutic tool but a life philosophy. It equips us with strategies to handle distress, regulate emotions, and build meaningful relationships. But more than that, it teaches us to be present, to accept, and to change. It's a compass that points to balance in all things.

3. The Ripple Effect of Recovery: Recovery from addiction doesn't just transform the individual; it has a ripple effect, touching every relationship, every interaction, and every moment. Stories of long-term sobriety successes aren't just tales of personal triumph; they're testaments to the transformative power of resilience, support, and self-awareness.

4. Self-Compassion as a Pillar of Strength: In our journey, we'll stumble. There will be moments of doubt, days of despair, and instances of relapse. But self-compassion teaches us to be our own ally. It's not about inflating our ego but about understanding our shared humanity. It's about recognizing that we're all works in progress, deserving of kindness, especially from ourselves.

5. Building Communities and Spreading Knowledge: Recovery is both a personal and communal journey. Sharing DBT with loved ones, building support groups, and advocating for mental health awareness creates a safety net. It fosters a community where everyone learns, grows, and heals together.

6. The Lifelong Nature of the Journey: Recovery isn't a destination but a continuous journey. Challenges in long-term sobriety remind us that growth is ongoing. Yet, with every challenge comes an opportunity: to learn, to adapt, and to become stronger.

7. The Role of Structure and Routine: As we've seen, structure provides a framework for recovery. Tailored routines, regular reflections, and clear goals provide a roadmap, guiding us through the complexities of life beyond addiction.

These takeaways are not just lessons but beacons, illuminating the path of recovery and personal growth. They remind us that every moment is an opportunity, every challenge a lesson, and every day a gift.

As we draw the curtains on this chapter, we find ourselves on the precipice of reflection, looking back at the vast landscape of knowledge, stories, and insights we've journeyed through. The tapestry of this book has been woven with threads of resilience, hope, and the transformative power of DBT. Each chapter, each story, each strategy has been a stepping stone, guiding us towards a deeper understanding of recovery and the profound impact of mindfulness and emotional regulation in our lives.

But every journey, no matter how enlightening, must find its moment of reflection, its point of culmination. As we prepare to turn the page to our concluding chapter, it's time to pause, breathe, and absorb the magnitude of what we've learned. The conclusion won't just be a summary; it will be a synthesis, a harmonious blend of every lesson, every challenge, and every triumph we've discussed.

In the next chapter, we'll take a step back to see the bigger picture. We'll connect the dots, revisiting the pivotal moments and key insights that have shaped our understanding. It's an opportunity to see how every piece fits together, forming a comprehensive guide to not just overcoming addiction, but truly living a life imbued with purpose, clarity, and joy. So, as we prepare to embark on this final leg of our journey, let's do so with gratitude, anticipation, and an open heart, ready to embrace the holistic wisdom that awaits.

# Chapter Eleven

---

# DBT: The Universal Tapestry of Transformation

As we dive into the world of education, imagine a classroom where students are not only equipped with academic knowledge but also tools to navigate their emotions. A place where a student struggling with anxiety can use DBT techniques to calm themselves before a big exam. The potential of DBT in schools is vast, and some pioneering institutions are already leading the way.

In the corporate realm, the pressures of modern work can often lead to burnout and emotional distress. But what if companies prioritized the emotional well-being of their employees as much as their quarterly profits? By integrating DBT into employee wellness programs, companies can foster a healthier, more productive work environment.

But the potential of DBT doesn't stop at schools and offices. Entire communities can be transformed by its principles. From local community centers offering DBT workshops to grassroots movements championing its benefits, the ripple effect is profound.

As we journey through this chapter, envision a future where DBT principles are interwoven into the very fabric of our society. A world where emotional well-being is a shared goal, and the principles of mindfulness, emotional regulation, and distress tolerance are common knowledge. This is the potential of a DBT-informed future, and it's a vision worth striving for.

**The Role of DBT in Shaping Societal Values:**

In the tapestry of society, individual threads, when woven together, create a collective fabric. Each thread, representing an individual's values, beliefs, and actions, contributes to the overall pattern. Now, imagine if a significant portion of these threads were imbued with the principles of DBT. The resulting societal fabric would be one of understanding, empathy, and resilience.

Historically, societies have been shaped by dominant ideologies, often influenced by political or religious beliefs. However, in the modern era, there's a growing recognition of the importance of emotional well-being and mental health. This shift is where DBT can play a pivotal role.

When individuals practice DBT, they not only enhance their own emotional intelligence but also influence those around them. Like a calming presence in a room full of chaos, a person grounded in DBT principles can subtly steer group dynamics towards understanding and collaboration. Over time, these individual actions can reshape societal norms, promoting values of empathy, patience, and open communication.

Moreover, as more people embrace DBT, there's a potential for societal structures to evolve. Imagine judicial systems that prioritize rehabilitation over punishment, or educational institutions that value emotional intelligence as much as academic prowess. The ripple effects of a DBT-informed populace can be profound and far-reaching.

**Pioneering a DBT Movement:**

The journey of a thousand miles begins with a single step. For those inspired by the transformative power of DBT, becoming an advocate can be that first step. But how does one person spark a movement?

It begins with personal conviction. By deeply internalizing DBT principles, individuals become living testimonials of its benefits. Their changed behaviors, improved relationships, and enhanced emotional well-being serve as tangible evidence of DBT's efficacy.

Next comes community engagement. Hosting local workshops, partnering with schools for awareness sessions, or even starting a DBT-themed podcast can spread the word. Collaborative efforts, such as joining hands with mental health professionals or community leaders, can amplify the reach.

However, pioneering a movement is not without challenges. Resistance from traditionalists, lack of resources, or personal setbacks can be disheartening. Yet, it's essential to remember the transformative stories of those who've benefited from DBT. Their journeys serve as a beacon, illuminating the path for others.

**The Future Vision of a DBT-Informed Society:**

As we stand on the cusp of a new era, the vision of a DBT-informed society beckons. But what might such a society look like?

Picture a world where emotional well-being is a shared priority. Schools, from elementary to universities, integrate DBT into their curriculums. Workplaces prioritize emotional health, with DBT workshops becoming as commonplace as team-building exercises.

In this envisioned society, technology plays a supportive role. Apps designed around DBT principles assist individuals in daily mindfulness practices. Virtual reality scenarios help people practice distress tolerance techniques in safe environments.

But beyond these tangible changes, the most profound transformation is in societal values. A DBT-informed society is one of understanding and empathy. Conflicts are approached with a desire for resolution rather than victory. Communities come together, not just in times of crisis but in daily life, fostering connections and mutual support.

DBT as a Universal Language:

In the vast expanse of human communication, there exists a myriad of languages, each with its unique syntax, grammar, and cultural nuances. Yet, despite the richness of our linguistic diversity, misunderstandings abound. Enter DBT, not as a spoken language, but as a universal language of understanding and empathy.

Imagine a scenario where two individuals, from vastly different backgrounds, find themselves in conflict. Their spoken languages might be different, their cultural references might not align, but if both are versed in the principles of DBT, a bridge of understanding can be built. Through the lens of mindfulness, they can approach the situation without judgment, focusing on the present moment. By employing distress tolerance techniques, they can navigate the emotional turbulence that often accompanies misunderstandings. And through effective communication strategies, they can articulate their perspectives, fostering mutual respect.

In a world that often feels fragmented, the principles of DBT offer a unifying thread. It's a language that transcends borders, cultures, and personal beliefs, focusing instead on our shared human experience. By embracing DBT as a universal language, we open the doors to deeper connections, not just with those in our immediate circles, but with humanity at large.

DBT and the Arts:

Art, in its many forms, has always been a reflection of society, capturing the zeitgeist of an era. From the intricate cave paintings of prehistoric times to the avant-garde movements of the 20th century, art tells a story. Now, imagine the infusion of DBT principles into the world of arts.

Visual artists, inspired by mindfulness, might create pieces that invite viewers to immerse themselves fully, experiencing the artwork in the present moment. Musicians might compose melodies that resonate with the rhythms of emotional regulation, offering solace to troubled souls. Writers, influenced by DBT's emphasis on interpersonal effectiveness, might craft narratives that delve deep into the complexities of human relationships.

Furthermore, the process of creating art can be therapeutic. Artists, by incorporating DBT techniques, can navigate the emotional highs and lows that often accompany the creative process. They can use distress tolerance techniques when faced with creative blocks, and employ mindfulness practices to stay grounded during moments of intense inspiration.

In this intertwining of DBT and the arts, we find a beautiful synergy. Art, with its ability to touch souls, combined with the transformative power of DBT, has the potential to usher in a renaissance of emotional well-being.

DBT's Legacy for Future Generations:

As we cast our gaze towards the horizon, pondering the legacy we wish to leave for future generations, the role of DBT becomes evident. It's not just a therapeutic approach for the present but a gift for the future.

Children, when introduced to DBT principles early in life, are equipped with tools that will serve them throughout their journey. They learn the value of emotional regulation, the importance of being present, and the skills to navigate the complexities of interpersonal relationships. These are not just lessons for a classroom but life skills that will stand them in good stead, whether they're facing academic challenges, navigating the tumultuous waters of adolescence, or stepping into the world as young adults.

Moreover, as these children grow and perhaps become parents themselves, they pass on these DBT principles to the next generation, creating a ripple effect. It's a legacy of emotional well-being, a gift that keeps on giving.

In the grand tapestry of human history, every generation leaves its mark. And as advocates of DBT, our mark is one of hope, resilience, and a deep understanding of the human experience. It's a legacy that speaks not just of personal healing but of a collective move towards a more empathetic and connected world.

In the vast tapestry of human experience, the principles of Dialectical Behavior Therapy (DBT) emerge as a beacon of hope, understanding, and transformation. As we journeyed through the final chapter of this enlightening book, several pivotal takeaways illuminated our path:

1. DBT as a Universal Language: Beyond the confines of therapy rooms and self-help books, DBT extends its reach as a universal language. It's not just a set of therapeutic techniques but a bridge that connects diverse individuals. By embracing the principles of mindfulness, distress tolerance, and effective communication, we can transcend linguistic barriers and cultural differences. In a world rife with misunderstandings, DBT offers a harmonizing tune, fostering connections that are deep, genuine, and lasting.

2. The Intersection of DBT and Art: Art, in all its myriad forms, has always mirrored society's soul. When DBT principles infuse the world of art, a transformative synergy arises. Artists, whether they paint, compose, or write, can channel the essence of DBT to create pieces that resonate with emotional depth. Moreover, the very act of creation becomes a therapeutic endeavor. Through DBT, artists find solace during creative blocks and remain grounded during whirlwinds of inspiration. The result? Art that not only pleases the senses but also heals the soul.

3. A Legacy for the Future: The seeds we plant today determine the fruits our future generations will reap. Introducing DBT to the younger generation is akin to equipping them with a compass for life.

The challenges of tomorrow might be unknown, but with DBT's principles, they'll have the tools to navigate any storm. Emotional regulation, mindfulness, and interpersonal effectiveness aren't just therapeutic jargon; they're life skills. And as these skills pass from one generation to the next, a legacy of emotional well-being and resilience takes shape.

4. The Ripple Effect: Every individual touched by DBT becomes a beacon for others. As they incorporate DBT into their daily lives, they inadvertently influence those around them. It's a ripple effect, where the transformation of one individual can lead to the collective growth of a community. Whether it's through direct advocacy or simply living the DBT principles, the impact is profound and far-reaching.

5. The Gift that Keeps on Giving: DBT isn't a one-time solution but a lifelong companion. As individuals evolve, so does their understanding and application of DBT. It's a gift that keeps on giving, offering insights, solace, and strategies at every life stage. From the tumultuous teenage years to the challenges of adulthood and the reflections of old age, DBT remains a steadfast ally.

In essence, this chapter illuminated the expansive potential of DBT. It's not confined to therapy sessions or specific challenges. Instead, its principles permeate every facet of life, offering insights, strategies, and hope.

As we close this enlightening chapter, our journey through the world of DBT doesn't end. Instead, it prepares us for the grand finale, where we'll weave together the threads of knowledge, insights, and experiences. The upcoming conclusion is not just a recapitulation but a celebration of the transformative power of DBT. It's a moment to reflect, rejoice, and recommit to a life enriched by the principles of Dialectical Behavior Therapy. So, let's embark on this final leg, cherishing the wisdom we've gained and anticipating the revelations that await.

# Conclusion

In the pages of this book, we've embarked on a transformative
journey, delving deep into the intricacies of addiction, recovery,
and the profound impact of Dialectical Behavior Therapy (DBT). We
began by understanding the very nature of addiction, its roots, and the
triggers that can lead to relapse. The importance of recognizing and
understanding these triggers was emphasized, as they play a pivotal
role in the recovery journey.

We then explored the world of DBT, a therapeutic approach that offers
tools and strategies to manage emotional distress, enhance self-awareness, and build resilience. Through various techniques, from mindfulness practices to emotional regulation, DBT provides a roadmap
to not just overcome addiction but to thrive in life.

Relationships, often strained by the weight of addiction, were also a
focal point. We delved into the challenges faced by those around the
addicted individual and the ways to rebuild trust and foster understanding. The significance of structure in recovery was highlighted,
showcasing how a well-defined structure can act as a protective shield
against potential relapses.

As we progressed, the broader applications of DBT in daily life challenges were unveiled. It's not just about addiction; it's about enhancing emotional intelligence, dealing with distress, and fostering personal growth. The journey of recovery is lifelong, and the stories of those who've walked this path before us serve as beacons of hope.

To every reader, know that the knowledge you've gained from this book is a powerful tool. But like any tool, its true potential is realized only when it's used. Embrace the strategies, practice the techniques, and lean into the wisdom shared. There will be challenges, moments of doubt, and times when the journey feels overwhelming. Yet, remember that every step you take, no matter how small, is a step towards a brighter, healthier, and more fulfilled life. The rewards of this journey, the peace, clarity, and joy, are truly worth every struggle.

Now, as you stand at this crossroad, the next step in your journey to a life of sobriety and emotional well-being is clear. Take action. Implement what you've learned, seek support, and be proactive in your recovery. Visualize a life where emotional turmoil is replaced with tranquility, where addiction's chains are broken, replaced by the freedom of self-awareness and control. I am here with you on this journey, committed to guiding, supporting, and cheering you on every step of the way. This is not just a book; it's a movement towards a better life. And your best life starts now.

Printed in Great Britain
by Amazon

35797260R00059